THE NURSES OF ELLIS ISLAND

THE NURSES OF ELLIS ISLAND
Life and Work inside the Golden Door

MICHELLE C. HEHMAN *and* ARLENE W. KEELING

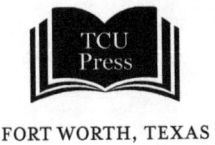

FORT WORTH, TEXAS

Cover

Ellis Island, Jersey City, New Jersey. Library of Congess, HS503-3068

Ellis Island nurse with immigrant children. National Park Service (Statue of Liberty National Monument)

Library of Congress Cataloging-in-Publication Data

Names: Hehman, Michelle C., author. | Keeling, Arlene Wynbeek, 1948– author.
Title: The nurses of Ellis Island : life and work inside the Golden Door /
    Michelle Hehman and Arlene Keeling.
Description: Fort Worth, Texas : TCU Press, [2024] | Includes bibliographical references and
    index. | Summary: "The Nurses of Ellis Island: Life and Work inside the Golden Door tells
    the story of the nurses who offered hope and healing to some of America's most vulnerable
    patients. In the once-modern hospital complex on the southwest side of Ellis Island, a
    small group of nurses from the U.S. Public Health Service expertly cared for more than
    150,000 patients of all ages and backgrounds, suffering from every imaginable illness
    and injury. These nurses, who lived and worked in the hospital built between the Main
    Immigration Building and the Statue of Liberty, learned to embrace their roles as both
    compassionate caregivers and agents of the state, all while navigating the impact of major
    sociopolitical events that included two world wars, a global pandemic, and increasingly
    restrictive immigration legislation. Drawing from government records, archival sources,
    and newly uncovered memoirs from the nurses themselves, award-winning authors and
    accomplished nurse historians Michelle Hehman and Arlene Keeling reconstruct the
    lived experience of nursing on Ellis Island during the first half of the twentieth century.
    This tale of nursing at its finest is a stunning narrative of triumph and tragedy that
    brings to life the largely invisible yet indispensable work of nursing at the intersection of
    immigration and public health policy"— Provided by publisher.
Identifiers: LCCN 2024041746 (print) | LCCN 2024041747 (ebook) |
    ISBN 9780875658889 (paperback) | ISBN 9780875658995 (ebook)
Subjects: LCSH: Ellis Island Hospital—History. | Public health nurses—Ellis Island (N.J. and
    N.Y.)—History. | Noncitizen detention centers—Health aspects—Ellis Island (N.J. and N.Y.)—
    History. | Immigrants—Medical care—United States—History—20th century.
Classification: LCC RT5.N4 H44 2024 (print) | LCC RT5.N4 (ebook) |
    DDC 610.7309747/1—dc23/eng/20240924
LC record available at https://lccn.loc.gov/2024041746
LC ebook record available at https://lccn.loc.gov/2024041747

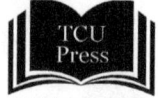

TCU Box 298300
Fort Worth, Texas 76129
www.tcupress.com

Design by Julie Rushing

*This book is dedicated to all of the nurses
who worked on Ellis Island.*

CONTENTS

ACKNOWLEDGMENTS

The idea for writing a history of nursing on Ellis Island came from our mentor and colleague Barbara Brodie, PhD, RN, FAAN, professor of nursing emerita at the University of Virginia and a "living legend" in the American Academy of Nursing. The project would never have happened had it not been for her lecture about what immigrants faced as they passed through Ellis Island on their way to the United States in the years 1892 to 1954. We thank Barbara for her interest in the book, for sharing with us her early archival notes, and for supporting our undertaking.

Several research trips to Ellis Island served to foster our interest in the nurses' story. A private hard hat tour of the abandoned hospitals on a freezing cold day in March 2017 not only allowed us to experience a choppy ferry commute from the Battery and the winds whipping off the water but also highlighted the fact that the nurses' story, for the most part, was invisible. After several years of research, we returned to the island in May 2019 with a more nuanced understanding of the immigrant hospitals but few details about the nurses' experiences. Hence our continued investigation to uncover them—a process that spanned several years.

Writing this history has been challenging, particularly for a lack of data. Early records (1892–1897) of the Ellis Island Hospital were destroyed when the first immigration station burned to the ground in 1897, and the whereabouts of the thousands of charts and other hospital records from 1902 and beyond remain unknown. That alone eliminated many of the potential primary sources for the years that nurses worked on Ellis Island. In addition, the fact that nurses typically did not document their own day-to-day work gave new meaning to the challenge of "making visible the invisible" in describing their work. For help in identifying and locating what primary data are still available, we would like to thank Barry Moreno, George Tselos, Matthew Housch, and the numerous National Park Service staff at the Bob Hope Memorial Library at Ellis Island, as well as archivists with the National Archives, both in the research room at College Park, Maryland, and those at the National Personnel Records Center in St. Louis, Missouri. Special recognition and gratitude go to Paul and Nina Bishop, the family of Margaret V. Daly, for their willingness to share Margaret's memoir and personal notes, help in tracing genealogy and verify timelines, and permission to tell Margaret's story.

We would like to thank Jim Peskin for his unwavering support of our research and for sharing his knowledge and resources to help us along the way. He was instrumental in facilitating our invitation to present an early version of this work as part of Save Ellis Island, Inc.,'s Virtual Author Series during the COVID-19 pandemic.

No history of nursing can be written without relying on multiple textbooks of nursing, and for sharing those sources, we acknowledge the Eleanor Crowder Bjoring Center for Nursing Historical Inquiry at the University of Virginia, the Barbara Bates Center for the Study of the History of Nursing at the University of Pennsylvania, and our colleagues from around the world for their publications on the history of nursing and healthcare.

A project of this magnitude requires funding and editing. Here, we must acknowledge the support of the Center for Nursing Research and the Global Center for Research at the University of Virginia, as well as funding from the 2017 Barbara Brodie Nursing History Fellowship from the Eleanor Crowder Bjoring Center for Nursing Historical Inquiry. We would also like to thank Doris Rikkers for serving as our managing editor, and the editorial staff at Texas Christian University Press for making their final review and publication of the manuscript.

Finally, our biggest thanks go to our families, friends, and colleagues for their love and support during the multiple years it took to complete this project. We would especially like to recognize Mike Hehman for his patience and wonderful sense of humor; Michael, Emma, and Matthew for being the best excuses to take a break from writing and for never complaining when Mom brought her work to basketball, volleyball, and baseball tournaments; Pat and Vicky Chambers for their constant encouragement; and Nicole Fontenot, Carliss Ramos, Joanne Muyco, and Alexis Hayes for listening, giving support, and offering to read drafts. We would also like to recognize Rich and Eric for providing a quiet and cozy place to write at their home on Cape Cod; Jenny, Gryphon, and L'Wren for Friday "pizza nights"; Amy, Owen, Macsen, and Avery for numerous FaceTime calls; and David, Jen, Zadie, and Auden for reminding us of what matters most.

INTRODUCTION

This book documents the history of nursing on Ellis Island from its opening in 1892 to its closure in 1954. Given the island's status as a national symbol of immigration and the "Golden Door" to the United States, most histories of Ellis Island have focused on preserving and highlighting the experience of the millions of immigrants who proceeded through the Great Hall on their way to becoming American citizens.[1] Nearly absent in those narratives, however, are stories about the nurses' work in the now-abandoned hospital buildings on the southwest section of the island. There, nurses and physicians provided state-of-the-art treatments to hundreds of thousands of patients, most of whom were newly arrived immigrants in need of medical attention after a long and sometimes harrowing journey across the Atlantic Ocean. Others were merchant marines and injured military men seeking care as government beneficiaries. Some, during World Wars I and II, were captured enemy aliens who were detained on the island. Nevertheless, regardless of race, culture, age, citizenship, or economic status, all the patients on Ellis Island were offered kindness, compassion, and clinical expertise by a small cadre of trained nurses. The powerful stories of these nurses have been largely neglected, left to fade alongside the deserted and crumbling wards of the once-modern hospital buildings. Indeed, the nurses' presence on the island—their life and work inside America's Golden Door—has been relegated to footnotes, a few artifacts, and old photographs. Until now.

Based on a wide variety of primary and secondary sources, the book tells the nurses' stories. Specifically, the book aims to (1) identify and describe the role of the nurses working at the hospital facilities on Ellis Island; (2) analyze how place, with varied definitions of the term, influenced the scope of the nurses' work and the delivery of care to hospitalized patients, particularly with respect to changes in federal immigration legislation; and (3) give voice to the Ellis Island nurses themselves.

The history of Ellis Island nurses—who they were, what they did, where they lived, and how they navigated their roles and responsibilities—centers on notions of *place*. Understanding how place takes a central role in the narrative is predicated on an analysis of the various definitions of the term. First, *place* encompasses the physical environment and surroundings in which the nurses practiced—two hospitals built on a tiny, mostly man-made island (technically three tiny islands linked together, first by small walkable bridges and later by landfill) in New York Harbor. *Place* also represents the particular period in time and the geopolitical and social context shaping the nurses' work. Another aspect of the term involves the designated role and status of Ellis Island nurses within their profession, within a racially segregated US society, and within the patriarchal medical hierarchy of the Marine Hospital Service in the late nineteenth century, and after 1902, the US Public Health Service (USPHS). Finally, *place* refers to a unique professional space for Ellis Island nurses, one in which they had to balance dual roles and competing responsibilities as both agents of the state and compassionate caregivers.

An assignment to Ellis Island meant living and working with a unique set of physical circumstances that could only be understood by those who experienced it. The geographical location of the island itself influenced those circumstances. The 27.5-acre island, located in New York Harbor between the coasts of New York and New Jersey, was a world unto itself, relying on the import of food and other necessities on a daily or weekly basis and the arrival of personnel and immigrants by ferryboat. While the nurses were stationed there, nearly every aspect of their lives was constrained by Ellis Island's geography. For nurses, this meant significant social isolation: they worked, ate, played, and slept on the island, only occasionally making the trip back to the mainland for recreation or necessity. Boundaries between the nurses' personal lives and professional identities all but disappeared; the demands of the job left little time for anything but work.

Another concept the book explores is "time as place." The time period in which Ellis Island nurses practiced was important. To help the reader understand the nurses' role on Ellis Island from 1892 to 1954, the book analyzes the scientific, social, and geopolitical context framing their experience. The influence of these factors becomes particularly apparent during World Wars I and II, when the scope of operations and duties of Ellis Island personnel changed altogether. During World War I, mass immigration from Europe slowed significantly and the island's focus changed from processing immigrants to processing American Red Cross Army nurses. Thus, the book includes the story of the army nurses who were stationed on Ellis Island for weeks to months at a time as they prepared to deploy to Europe—caught between their civilian life in the United States and the frontlines in France an ocean away. From late June 1917 to the spring of 1918, nurses were not only subjects to be processed themselves but also agents of the government, taking care of wounded and sick US soldiers returning to the island's hospitals and witnessing the activities of German internees. During World War II, the Ellis Island nurses' roles and duties shifted once again; they cared for coastguardsmen and their families stationed on the island, interned German, Italian, and Japanese enemy aliens, and a trickle of European immigrants.

Nurses' professional *place* within the prevailing medical hierarchy in general, within the USPHS hierarchy in particular, and within the patriarchal social and racial structures of the era also influenced nursing practice on Ellis Island. The book highlights the fact that nurses working on the island were expected to navigate in a "middle place," straddling the social expectations of their class and gender within the confines of a complex military-style, government-controlled, and racially segregated medical system, all while remaining true to their nursing code of ethics and professional responsibilities. Indeed, the nurses were "ordered to care"; they were expected to be obedient and self-sacrificing while ensuring that their patients received competent and compassionate treatment.[2]

Finally, *place* refers to the unique professional position from which the Ellis Island nurses provided care. In 1891 Congress took control of immigration laws and used the threat of communicable disease to justify medical deportations, thus creating an explicit link between federal immigration restrictions and public health policies. As employees of the USPHS, the nurses on Ellis Island practiced within this intersection, their duties as caregivers to individual patients overlapping with their commitment to uphold immigration laws in an effort to guard the health of the nation. Learning to navigate these sometimes-conflicting responsibilities became the most challenging aspect of the nurses' work at the most famous gateway to the United States, especially when they cared for immigrant patients with mandatory excludable conditions. In these cases, protecting the health of the American public meant destroying the hopes of an immigrant and their family.

Thus, it is through this framework of *place*, with multiple interpretive lenses, that the book tells the history of nursing on Ellis Island. Employing a unique style, the book incorporates elements of narrative nonfiction into a more traditional historical account in order to reconstruct the Ellis Island nurses' lived experiences.[3] This method, also referred to as "creative nonfiction," uses an informal tone that allows readers to make stronger connections to the nurses' individual experiences. The nurses are identified by their full names at first mention, and then only by their first names thereafter, just as they would have identified themselves and their peers. In contrast, physicians are addressed by their titles and last names, the same way that Ellis Island nurses would have addressed them professionally. In this book, that naming system was as much a necessity as it was a choice, since nearly all primary and secondary sources identified USPHS physicians using only initials for their first names. That said, the stories of the nurses' life and work presented here are based on valid and reliable primary sources, including Margaret Daly's memoir and official USPHS employment record, American Red Cross nurses' diaries from university and hospital archives, transcripts of interviews from the Oral History Project overseen by the Ellis Island National Museum of Immigration, and records of the United States Public Health Service and Immigration Service from the National Archives and Records Administration (College Park Campus). Sources also include articles from nursing journals of the 1890s to the 1950s, archival government reports, newspaper articles, and records from the archives on Ellis Island itself.

Following the chronologic history of Ellis Island as an immigration station and military depot from 1892–1954, the book is divided into six chapters, each with a discrete timeframe and central theme. Specifically:

CHAPTER 1, "Nurses on Ellis Island in the Early Years, 1892–1901," begins with a *New York Times* report on the opening of the new federal Ellis Island Immigration Station in 1892. Written from the point of view of the *New York Times* reporter, the chapter then describes the need for federal government control of immigration after the passage of the Immigration Act of 1891 and in response to the corruption in Castle Garden, the previous site for immigrant inspection. The chapter includes a description of the small forty-bed hospital on the island, the nurses' daily routines, and the problems of epidemics in the late nineteenth century. Also included is a brief description of the nurses' efforts to save patients when fire broke out at the Ellis Island Immigration Station and spread to the hospital in 1897, destroying most of the original buildings and the records stored in them. (Because of the loss of records, this chapter relies on nursing journals of the era and newspaper accounts for source material.) The chapter ends by mentioning the temporary return of immigration activities to the Battery in Manhattan while a newer station was being built. In 1900 the new Ellis Island Immigration Station opened, and, after lengthy delays, in 1902 a new general hospital was ready to accept patients on Island 2.

CHAPTER 2, "Caring for the Huddled Masses, 1902–1911," opens with the hiring of Margaret V. Daly as one of the first trained nurses to work for the Ellis Island General Hospital, describing her arrival and initial activities from her point of view. The chapter then provides a description of the inspection process to which immigrants were subjected and the nurses' role in their care if and when they were admitted to the hospital. It discusses the nurses' work on the wards, outlining their responsibilities and analyzing their interactions with immigrant patients and families. The chapter includes a description of the education and characteristics of Ellis Island nurses, as well as a depiction of the challenges they faced providing round-the-clock care, seven days a week, to thousands of poverty-stricken, non-English-speaking immigrants. It also provides an overview of the difficulties nurses encountered while caring for patients on Ellis Island and the ways they learned to manage and overcome these challenges. The chapter concludes with a discussion of the impact of contagious illness on the newly arrived immigrants and the need to construct appropriate isolation and treatment facilities on the island.

CHAPTER 3, "Nursing in the Contagious Disease Hospital, 1911–1917," opens with Chief Nurse Margaret Daly inspecting the buildings of the newly built Contagious Disease Hospital on Island 3 to ensure their readiness to receive patients. It goes on to describe the new hospital, emphasizing the thoughtful architectural design of the buildings and the detailed procedures nurses employed to prevent the spread of infectious disease from one ward to another. The chapter describes the nursing care of patients with different infectious diseases (including measles, favus, and trachoma), along with an analysis of the difficulties the nurses faced as they cared for immigrants diagnosed with mandatory excludable conditions. These patients, more than any other, presented the nurses with the challenge of balancing their role as caring professionals with that of being federal employees tasked with protecting the health of the public. The chapter concludes with changes taking place on Ellis Island as the United States entered World War I in April 1917. By June of that year, the island would become a mobilization center for Red Cross Army nurses.

CHAPTER 4, "Nurses on Ellis Island during World War I, 1917–1919," opens with a discussion of the changes Chief Nurse Margaret Daly observed in the Ellis Island General Hospital as she walked through the wards in June 1917. That month, German prisoners and US coastguardsmen were among the patients filling the wards of the General Hospital. The chapter then transitions to an account from the perspective of army nurse Edith Mury as she ferried to Ellis Island. Her new assignment was to oversee Red Cross Army nurses sent there for mobilization prior to being deployed to Europe. Based on primary source data from newly enlisted Red Cross Army nurses, the chapter addresses the experience of young civilian registered nurses being prepared for military service abroad. The chapter also discusses the US Army's takeover of the Ellis Island hospitals less than a year later in March 1918, sparking the end of Red Cross nurse mobilization on Ellis Island and the reassignment of Margaret Daly to Stapleton Hospital on Staten Island. The chapter concludes with Daly's 1919 return to Ellis Island as chief nurse after the war; the nurses' attempts to cope with the 1918 influenza pandemic; and the return of immigrants to the island hospitals in the 1920s.

CHAPTER 5, "Changing Rules and Changing Roles, 1920–1939," explores the impact of World War I on immigration and the hospital activities on Ellis Island. Beginning with a discussion of surgical nursing, the chapter goes on to describe the sociopolitical atmosphere of the United States, particularly with respect to federal immigration legislation after the war. The passage of the 1921 and 1924 Immigration Acts, initiating the national origins quota program and consular control system that would effectively end the era of mass immigration, transformed all activities on the island. These new laws had an immediate impact on the types of patients admitted to Ellis Island hospitals in the 1920s and 1930s. Now more marine servicemen rather than immigrants occupied the hospital beds, the change altering the character and rhythm of the nurses' work. During this period, nursing responsibilities increased while the hospital census declined in the wake of severe immigration restrictions. The chapter offers a detailed look at the work nurses did as they assisted with more complex surgeries, cared for detained immigrants suffering from contagious illness, and struggled to meet the demands of increasing psychiatric and tuberculosis cases among Marine Hospital Service beneficiaries. The chapter ends with the creation of a United States Coast Guard base on the island when war again broke out in Europe in 1939.

CHAPTER 6, "World War II and the End of a Nursing Presence on Ellis Island, 1941–1954," covers nursing on Ellis Island from the WWII years to the island's closure in the mid-1950s. It discusses the use of Ellis Island as an Alien Enemy Internment Camp during the war and the implications of those changes for nursing. It goes on to review the decline in hospital admissions due to increasingly restrictive immigration policies after the war and the events that led to the closing of the hospital in 1951 and of all facilities on the island in November 1954. The chapter ends with a reexamination of the contributions that the nurses made during their time on Ellis Island, focusing on the importance of documenting their legacy of care.

In addition to highlighting the essential role of nurses on Ellis Island and giving voice to those nurses, the narrative reveals the enduring nature of many issues surrounding immigration, public health, and the role of nurses in society. The story offers yet another example of nurses serving vulnerable and marginalized communities and offering compassion and expert care to their patients while navigating complex social and political environments, changing physical environments and procedures, and challenging directives from those in authority. It is a story that is ongoing and will likely continue, as the US government faces an immigration emergency at the nation's southern border and anticipates a worsening global refugee crisis in the future.

Nurse participation in policy planning for the healthcare needs of migrants and refugees is essential given their unique perspective on the front line of care. Evidence from nursing history can inform and direct policy development, as it documents how nurses have worked to provide quality care to vulnerable populations in the past and have served as advocates for the compassionate and dignified care for all people who seek freedom and opportunity in the United States.

Michelle C. Hehman
Arlene W. Keeling

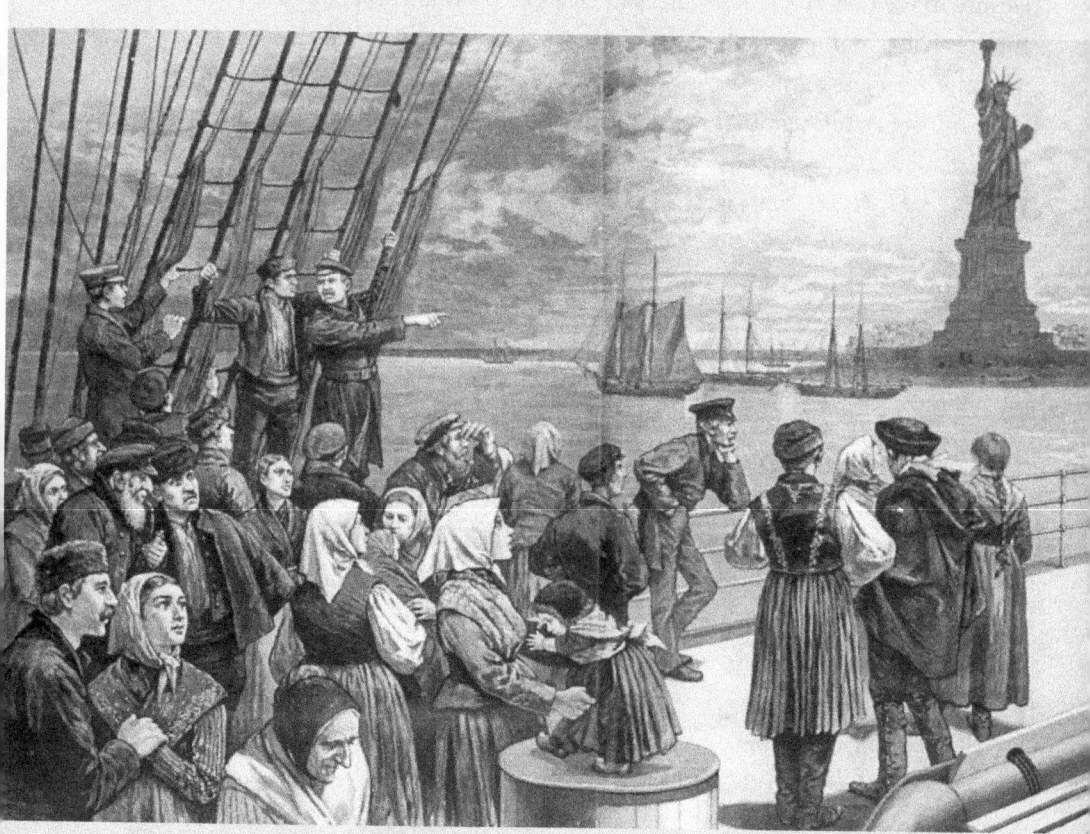
Illustration of immigrants on the deck of a steamship passing the Statue of Liberty, 1887.
Courtesy of the Library of Congress, Prints and Photographs Online Catalog.

CHAPTER 1

NURSES ON ELLIS ISLAND IN THE EARLY YEARS 1892–1901

LANDED ON ELLIS ISLAND
New Immigration Buildings
Opened Yesterday

A Rosy-Cheeked Irish Girl the
First Registered. Room Enough
for All Arrivals

NEW YORK TIMES, JANUARY 2, 1892[1]

Waiting for the first transport barge to land on Ellis Island, the *New York Times* journalist pulled his scarf a little higher, wishing he had worn a heavier coat.[2] His latest assignment had brought him to the tiny island in New York Harbor on this frigid New Year's Day to cover the opening of the new federal Immigration Building. Now, bracing himself against the bitter winds coming off the bay, he shivered alongside the rest of the reporters standing on the wharf. At least he could see the *John E. Moore* making its way across the bay.[3] The barge, bringing passengers from the steamship *Nevada*, was due to land in about ten more minutes. Then, perhaps he could follow the immigrants and the receiving party inside the station, where it would be warmer.

Looking around, he took note of the new building and the people he needed to mention in his article. First, he noted the three government officials who stood on the wharf to greet the arriving immigrants. Colonel John B. Weber, the superintendent of immigration, was, of course, front and center. Standing next to Weber was Major George Hibbard, the superintendent of construction for the Ellis Island facility, and Surgeon George W. Stoner, the physician assigned to Ellis Island.[4] Flexing his ice-cold fingers, the reporter jotted down the three names; they all deserved mention. Continuing to scan the welcoming party, he saw that the three dignitaries were not alone. Toward the back stood numerous Ellis Island staff members, including railroad men, baggage handlers, cooks, and a small group of nurses.[5] Too many to name, he thought, but then again, the nurses did add a bit of color to the scene with their long cotton uniforms and woolen capes whipping in the wind. Maybe he should include them; maybe not.

Ah, here came the ferry now. A clang of bells and "a din of shrieking whistles" heralded its arrival.[6] Scribbling down details in his tiny notebook, the journalist turned his attention to those disembarking. He noted a fair-skinned, rosy-cheeked girl, accompanied by two younger boys, skipping down the gangplank. With that hair and skin coloring, they had to be Irish, he thought. He would need to get the girl's name and the facts about the specific country she had sailed from. No doubt they'd fit the perfect description of all the other Irish immigrants who had been seeking opportunity in America since the mid-nineteenth century.[7]

Next, he took notes describing the massive new immigration station. He made sure to highlight that the new reception building had "room enough" to accommodate the almost seven thousand European immigrants anticipated to arrive at Ellis Island every day.[8] He also drew attention to the facts that the new structure had a large baggage area, a huge reception hall for inspections, and even a hospital for those who were sick.

Jotting down details as quickly as possible, the reporter described the opening ceremonies, focusing on how Colonel Weber presented the girl with a ten-dollar gold piece for being the first to land at the new immigration station on Ellis Island. He wrote down the particulars of the luncheon for the dignitaries and the Ellis Island staff that followed, noted the speed in which passengers were processed in the new station, and listed the names of the ships on which they had sailed for the United States. Of the seven hundred immigrants who registered that day, some had arrived on the steamship *Nevada*, others on the *City of Paris* and the *Victoria*.[9]

Half-frozen fingers notwithstanding, the reporter concluded this assignment had been worth it—the story would make for a great column. Of course, it still needed work but at least he had discovered more details about the first immigrant girl to be registered. Her name was Annie Moore and she and her two younger brothers had traveled from County Cork, Ireland, to join their parents already in the United States. The ceremonies being over, the reporter returned to the mainland to file his story before his midnight deadline. It had to make the morning paper!

News of the new immigration building on Ellis Island spread rapidly throughout the country, as newspapers in major cities and in small towns across America picked up the story. Most of the articles focused on the "little Irish lass"—"the first immigrant to land on Federal ground"—while others reported that "the entire population of the Island" cheered Annie's arrival.[10] As was true of the initial *New York Times* report, notably absent from the coverage was any description of the "entire population" of Ellis Island—the watchmen, baggage handlers, and railway ticket clerks who worked behind the scenes, or the nurses, cooks, ward maids, and apothecary who cared for immigrant patients in the small hospital behind the Great Hall.

Of the "entire population," the nurses were particularly important to immigrants who were not as healthy as Annie and her brothers when they arrived. While the energetic Irish girl and her younger brothers breezed through the health inspection process, other passengers did not. Some were detained for further inspection. Others were quite sick when they landed and needed hospitalization. The nurses, cooks, ward maids, and the apothecary were all essential to managing their care. Of these, the nurses were indispensable, not only because they provided direct physical care but also because they often stepped in to manage the diet kitchen, clean the wards, or fill medication bottles when those responsible for the tasks were absent or simply needed an extra pair of hands.

NEW POLICIES: THE IMMIGRATION ACT OF 1891

Another piece of information missing in the news coverage was the fact that Annie and her brothers were poor and had traveled in the ship's steerage class. This was the only class of passengers now required to pass through medical inspection lines on Ellis Island. Just a few months earlier Congress had passed the Immigration Act of 1891, changing the immigration process. Now in the hands of the *federal* government, the new process was described in *Harper's Weekly*:

> Steerage passengers would be loaded off barges at Ellis Island and ascend to the second-story for medical inspection and interrogation. Some would be detained for further physical examination; the others will continue into the great second-story room, to be separated into ten lines and to

march through that number of aisles between the desks of the so-called "pedigree clerks," who will cross-examine them as the law requires.[11]

The same law mandated that first- and second-class passengers be inspected in their cabins aboard ship. Unless they showed signs of a contagious disease, they would disembark and proceed directly into the United States.[12] The changes made by the Immigration Act of 1891 were significant, breaking with previous state immigration policies and arrival procedures.

ARRIVAL PROCEDURES BEFORE THE IMMIGRATION ACT OF 1891

Prior to 1891, each state had been in charge of immigration policies for its own ports. In New York, all noncontagious immigrants, including steerage-class passengers, were ferried from the ships on which they arrived in the harbor to the wharf at the Battery on the tip of Manhattan. As many as three thousand immigrants disembarked directly onto the mainland every day. Having made their way down the gangplank, the newcomers proceeded through Castle Garden's circular sandstone fort, where they received a cursory health inspection by *state* officials. If they passed, they were free to go on their way; if not, they were detained for further evaluation. Some were deported.

The immigrants who traveled in first- and second-class cabins (indicating that they were from the upper or middle class) and those who could speak English usually had no problems making their way through the state health inspection. However, poor immigrants who traveled in the steerage compartment and those who could not understand English faced numerous problems during their time in the corrupt environment of Castle Garden.

For decades con artists preyed on newcomers unfamiliar with American customs, money, and language. Swindlers demanded exorbitant payments for such services as locating boarding houses, "guarding" the immigrants' baggage, exchanging money, or purchasing railway tickets to various destinations across the country. As Joseph Pulitzer's newspaper, the *World*, described it, Castle Garden was "a place of tyranny and whimsical rule, a place for the abuse and insult of helpless women, for the inhuman treatment of mothers and children . . . [and] for the privation of the poor."[13] Moreover, instead of addressing these issues, New York State officials, under the control of the corrupt bosses of Tammany Hall, looked the other way. Now, with the Immigration Act of 1891, the federal government showed itself determined to deal with that corruption.

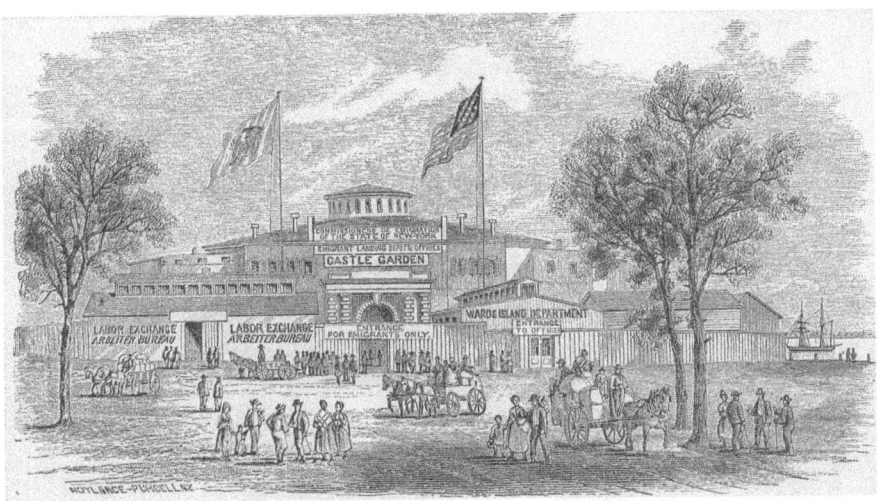

Illustration of the New York state emigrant landing depot at Castle Garden, circa 1861–1880.
Courtesy of the Miriam and Ira D. Wallach Picture Collection, New York Public Library Digital Collections

AN EXCEPTION TO FEDERAL CONTROL: QUARANTINE PROCEDURES

After 1891 state quarantine procedures varied throughout the country. In New York, state authorities, having refused to fully relinquish their role to federal agents, continued to control the quarantine procedures. As had been the case in previous years, international steamships carrying immigrants remained offshore to await a quarantine evaluation before being permitted to dock. State health officials then boarded the newly arrived ships to inspect the immigrants, identified those with symptoms of serious "germ diseases," and took them to the quarantine station on Hoffman Island or to the hospital on Swinburne Island (both in operation since 1872). There the sick passengers were kept in quarantine under state health officials' control.[14] When considered healthy, the immigrants were sent to Ellis Island, where Marine Hospital Service physicians, employed by the federal government, screened them further before granting them access to the United States or sending them back to their home countries.

A NEW STATION FOR MEDICAL INSPECTION

The new facility on Ellis Island, built by the federal government at a cost of five hundred thousand dollars, was large enough to "easily process 7,000 immigrants" a day.[15] An 1891 article in *Harper's Weekly* extolled the architecture of the new station, describing it as "a latter-day watering place hotel" complete with "a great many-windowed expanse of buff-painted wooden walls, of blue-slate roofing, and of light and picturesque towers."[16] Indeed, the author went on, the new station's modern architecture signaled how different it would be from Castle Garden—"putting to shame" the conditions in which "neglectful State officials" had "previously mismanaged the business."[17]

The primary function of that "business" was the medical inspection of immigrants. During that process, Marine Hospital Service physicians (later USPHS physicians) were tasked with identifying anyone who suffered from a condition that required mandatory exclusion and deportation under the 1891 Immigration Act. These conditions included "loathsome" diseases like leprosy and venereal disease. In addition, a diagnosis of insanity or idiocy—or any condition that increased the likelihood of the patient's becoming a public charge—required immediate deportation.[18] Any immigrant who was not "clearly and beyond a doubt entitled to land" would be temporarily held for further investigation, to await a hearing before the Board of Special Inquiry.[19]

Immigrants needing medical treatment were sent to the newly constructed forty-bed "model" hospital located just behind the main reception building.[20] There, a Marine Hospital Service physician and three nurses, along with ward maids, cooks, and an apothecary, provided care.[21] Of these, the nurses played a major role, caring for patients twenty-four hours a day, seven days a week.

THE ELLIS ISLAND NURSES

Had the *New York Times* reporter interviewed the nurses on that opening day, he would have discovered that the three nurses staffing the original Ellis Island Hospital shared one important characteristic that was as noteworthy of headlines as the new immigration station itself. All three were women who had completed at least some formal nurses' training or had years of hospital nursing experience. That characteristic set them apart from nursing staff in other hospitals in the country. The Ellis Island Hospital was not affiliated with a nurse training school, so unlike other US hospitals that typically relied on pupils from their training programs to staff the wards, Ellis Island Hospital could not turn to student nurses for help.[22] Hiring experienced nurses was clearly the only way to staff the hospital, and by 1892 several New York City hospital-based training schools were prepared to supply them. These schools included the famous Training School for Nurses at Bellevue Hospital (opened in 1873), Mt. Sinai's Training School for Nurses (opened

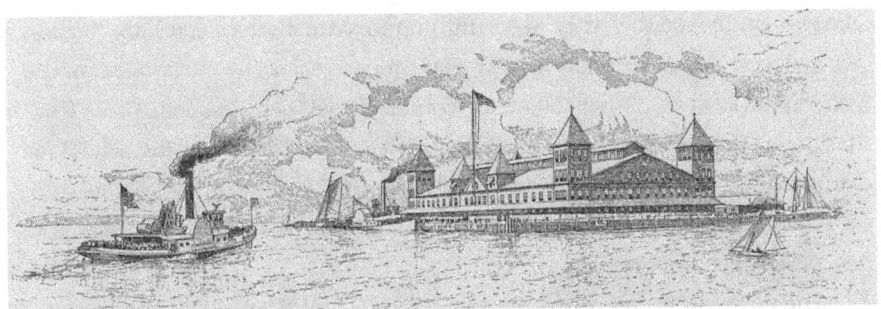

Illustration of the Ellis Island immigrant building, 1891.
Courtesy of the Miriam and Ira D. Wallach Picture Collection, New York Public Library Digital Collections.

in 1881), the Maternity and Charity Hospital Training School on Blackwell Island (opened in 1886), and St. Luke's Hospital Training School (opened in 1888).[23] In addition, graduate nurses from hospitals elsewhere in the country were recruited to work for the Marine Hospital Service.

Besides being experienced, the nurses employed on Ellis Island in the 1890s were almost by default White.[24] Some were of Irish or German descent, others Dutch or eastern European. In the 1890s, on the East Coast of the United States, none were Asian or Native American; neither were they Black. In the racially segregated US society of 1892, only a handful of Black graduate nurses were available for hire—even if a concerted effort had been made to employ them. By 1889 only six Black women had graduated from the New England Hospital for Women and Children in Boston, one of the few northern schools that accepted Black students on a strict annual quota system. Moreover, in 1892 very few Black women had matriculated through the only two nurse training schools in the United States specifically designated for them: Provident Hospital in Chicago and the Dixie Hospital Training School in Hampton, Virginia. The Tuskegee Institute opened a nurse training course for Black nursing students in 1892 but it would take at least two years for that school to produce graduates. A few other schools for Black nursing students opened later in the decade—mostly in the South, where many of their graduates remained.[25] The scarcity of available Black nurses for hire was not the main issue, however. Regrettably, in America's racially segregated society of the 1890s, the Marine Hospital Service officials did not even consider hiring a Black nurse.

In addition to their experience and their race, the Ellis Island nurses most likely shared another characteristic: they were from the working or middle classes. Quite possibly they were immigrants themselves, perhaps having arrived as children a few decades earlier. In part, their class depended on the geographic location of their hometown or the school they attended. Those from Boston area schools, with the exception of the elite Boston Training School for Nurses, were often working class; those from New York training schools were usually middle-class women who had previously worked as teachers, secretaries, saleswomen, or governesses.[26]

The nurses who accepted work at the Ellis Island Hospital also had several other traits in common. First, they needed the work and preferred to work as a staff nurse in a hospital rather than as a private-duty nurse in someone's home. Second, they were well-disciplined, "cool, competent, and courageous" professionals who accepted their "gendered place within a hierarchal medical structure."[27] Third, having accepted employment in the Marine Hospital Service, the nurses were agents of the federal government and expected to uphold the immigration laws of the United States. Finally, the nurses were accountable to the Marine Hospital Service physicians, who were in turn accountable to the surgeon general. A document from the office of the surgeon general outlined the "quasi military character" of that service:

> The organization is of a military character. . . . Many of the officers . . .
> are members of the Association of Military Surgeons of the United States
> under constitutional provisions of that body. . . . All officers are subject
> by law and regulations to the orders of the Surgeon-General of the
> Marine Hospital Service.[28]

Clearly, the nurses working in this "quasi-military" medical establishment, carrying out physicians' medical orders, were themselves subject to the surgeon general's laws and regulations. Together, these features would determine how the nurses implemented care in the small Ellis Island Hospital.

INVISIBLE BUT INDISPENSABLE

Despite the fact that the Ellis Island nurses were invisible in the news coverage of the island's opening, they were indispensable to patients and physicians alike. Patients needed care; physicians needed assistance. Of the thousands of steerage-class passengers coming through Ellis Island each day, some were certain to suffer from acute diseases like pneumonia, bronchitis, or thyroiditis, while others had chronic medical conditions like psychiatric disorders, heart failure, or kidney disease. Pregnant women were sometimes close to their delivery date when they arrived. Small children presented with gastrointestinal illnesses acquired during the time they spent in the cramped and unsanitary conditions of the ships' steerage quarters. Moreover, weeks of seasickness and paltry rations of "decaying herring, rotten potatoes [and] stale black bread" added to the likelihood that many poverty-stricken immigrants arrived dehydrated and malnourished, further complicating their medical conditions.[29]

Winding their way through the second-floor reception hall after landing on Ellis Island, immigrants received cursory medical inspections. Those who passed the examination made their way back downstairs to the railroad ticket counters and ferries to the mainland. Others, marked for further evaluation, were held in detention rooms. Those deemed too sick to travel were sent to the Ellis Island Hospital. There, graduate nurses, dressed in immaculate, ankle-length cotton uniforms covered with starched white aprons, provided the patients with round-the-clock care, working "practically on continuous duty, no exceptions being made with regard to Sundays or legal holidays."[30]

In the hospital, the nurses followed specific Marine Hospital guidelines and physicians' orders to implement care. In addition, they relied on what they had learned in school to carry out specific treatments and manage the ward environment.[31] They sought advice from books like *Notes on Hospitals*, published in 1859 by the famous British nurse Florence Nightingale. They also turned to articles from the *Trained Nurse and Hospital Review*, the leading nursing journal in the United States in the 1890s.

THE ELLIS ISLAND HOSPITAL: THE IMPORTANCE OF PLACE

The setting in which the nurses worked was important to the results they could achieve. The new hospital, located just behind the Great Hall in the Main Immigration Building, was composed of a group of one- and two-story wooden buildings with sheltered verandas, arranged on a quadrangular plan around a central courtyard. The building was made of Georgia pine; the interior finished in natural wood.[32]

The hospital was a state-of-the-art facility, mirroring the pavilion model recommended by Florence Nightingale. As such, the Ellis Island Hospital avoided the three main "defects" that Nightingale believed contributed to increased mortality in hospitals: deficiencies of space, light, and ventilation.[33] In contrast, the Ellis Island Hospital had all three in abundance. Adequately spaced iron beds lined two sides of the wards. Large windows let in plenty of sunlight and could be opened to capture breezes off the harbor, providing the wards with ventilation far exceeding that of inner-city hospitals. Moreover, the central courtyard lined with verandas provided patients the opportunity to sit outside, protected from "wind, rain, or sun," while they took advantage of the "healing powers of light" and an abundance of fresh air.[34]

GENERAL NURSING CARE AT THE ELLIS ISLAND HOSPITAL

Working in the forty-bed hospital, Ellis Island nurses cared for immigrants using state-of-the-art scientific knowledge as the basis for their care. In 1892 nurses and physicians on Ellis Island adhered to the germ theory of disease, postulated by the German bacteriologist Robert Koch in 1876 with his discovery of the bacteria that caused anthrax. That theory had been further supported in 1882 with Koch's discovery of the organism responsible for tuberculosis, and in 1883 with his discovery of the germ that caused cholera.[35] Thus, as historian David Rosner explains, by 1892 both physicians and nurses recognized the germ theory's "simplicity, usefulness and cohesiveness" and incorporated it into "older sanitarian notions regarding the relationship between cleanliness, godliness and health."[36]

In the Ellis Island Hospital of the 1890s, the physicians and nurses also adopted the principles of antisepsis and asepsis. Twenty-five years earlier, the British surgeon Joseph Lister had published the results of his study on the treatment of wound infections using carbolic acid dressings. Following Lister's advice, the nurses not only used these dressings on patients' wounds but also washed their hands with carbolic acid soap and water provided by the island's large cistern. Moreover, they sprayed the operating room with carbolic acid prior to a surgery and assisted surgeons using aseptic technique—scrubbing before surgery, donning sterile gowns, and using instruments that had been autoclaved.[37]

The equipment the nurses used at Ellis Island Hospital was also state-of-the-art. They bathed sick children in porcelain-enameled iron bathtubs, fed patients using spouted ceramic cups, moved patients from place to place using wooden wheelchairs and iron gurneys, placed newborn infants in wicker bassinets, and weighed both children and adults on white enamel scales.[38] Using the latest

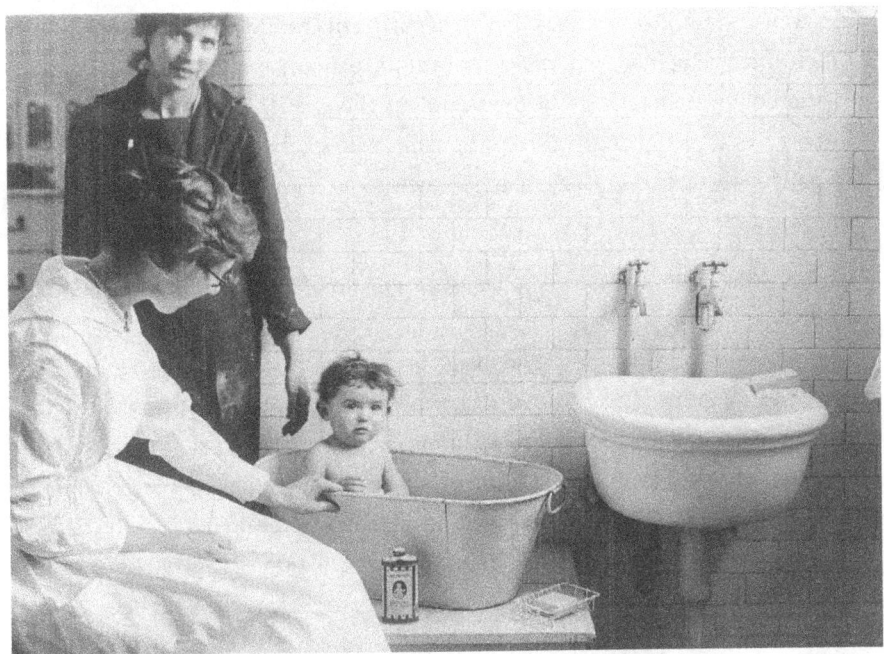

Nurse maid bathing infant patient in the Ellis Island hospital.
Courtesy of the National Park Service, Statue of Liberty National Monument.

technology available at the time, the nurses took their patients' temperatures with leading-edge six-inch glass thermometers. Designed by Thomas Albutt in 1866, the small mercury thermometers provided an accurate reading in just five minutes, a welcome alternative to the old foot-long instrument that required twenty minutes to register a patient's temperature.[39]

The Ellis Island nurses observed patients carefully for any indication of a change in their condition. During their training programs, nurses had been taught the importance of making close observations and carefully recording them. As historian Margarete Sandelowski described that training, "Nurses were taught to cultivate their senses for the close observation that made nursing a scientific profession as opposed to a merely mechanical practice."[40]

The importance of the nurses' role in patient observation was emphasized repeatedly in the *Trained Nurse and Hospital Review*. Writing in the March 1896 issue, Dr. Anna Fullerton expressed her thoughts on the matter:

> The physician's time must of necessity be taken up with study and
> research; in other words, the planning of the campaign against any

given disease. To affect the purpose of curing his patient, he must have a trained helper: one who can remain at the patient's bedside, who thoroughly understands the physician's method and purposes; who observes to the letter all his requirements; whose careful records of a patient's condition will lead to the immediate application of remedies indicated.[41]

In other words, the nurse was to be an extension of the physician's mind and hands.[42]

Implementing what they had been taught, nurses not only checked the patient's temperature but also noted changes in their skin color, turgor, and the presence of rashes or petechiae. In addition, they counted the patient's pulse and observed the number and depth of their respirations.[43] Following the guidelines to "record the temperature of a patient immediately after taking it" and adding an accurate report of the pulse and respirations, the nurses kept careful charts of the information they obtained and reported any significant changes to the physician.[44] "More importantly," as historian Patricia D'Antonio has argued, "nurses' knowledge allowed them to understand the implications of the resulting data. . . . Nurses would follow orders—but not mindlessly or rigidly."[45]

In the late nineteenth century, few specific pharmacologic agents existed that were targeted directly at the underlying cause of the illness. As was true elsewhere, medical care and nursing care on Ellis Island overlapped significantly. Providing patients with a clean bed in a well-ventilated room, administering nutritious foods and fluids, bathing them to reduce fever, positioning them to prevent bedsores, and applying splints and bandages were key components of both medical and nursing care. The nurses had been drilled on how to provide these essentials. Using that knowledge, they took actions to alleviate the patients' symptoms and promote their comfort. For example, prior to the discovery of aspirin, nurses used sponge baths not only to reduce body temperature but also to "quiet the nerves and induce sleep."[46]

Before intravenous solutions were used for rehydration, nurses gave patients fluids and nutrients by mouth. For example, "toast water" was often given to treat dehydration and fever. According to an article in the *Trained Nurse and Hospital Review*, the recipe for toast water was simple: "Cut half a slice of stale bread, toast it thoroughly, and put it into a jug. Boil a quart of water. . . . Cool, and then pour it over the bread. A little lemon or orange peel may be added."[47]

Like other nurses practicing in the 1890s, Ellis Island nurses gave their patients other nutritious beverages, including cocoa, milk punch, linseed tea, egg brandy, barley water, buttermilk, soda water, soup, and beef broth.[48] All of these were given on a strict schedule, just as the nurses had been taught. As one nurse described the routine, "At 11:00 [a.m.] tonics are given out, afterwards eggnogs and milk punches are made and distributed."[49] Sometimes the nurses administered a "pinch of salt in a cup of hot water" to rehydrate a patient, or "beef jelly" to provide protein.[50] Egg brandy was particularly useful for "cases of prostration."[51] According to a recipe in the *Trained Nurse and Hospital Review*, the nurse was to "take the whites and yolks of three eggs and beat them up in five ounces of plain water. Add three ounces of brandy slowly, also add a little sugar and nutmeg" and administer it "two tablespoonfuls at a time."[52]

For the most part, the medications the Ellis Island nurses dispensed were directed toward symptom relief. Among the drugs most frequently prescribed were morphine, codeine, laudanum, Listerine, castor oil, bicarbonate of soda, Frazer's migraine, soda mint, calomel, syrup of ipecac, digitalis leaf, paregoric, tablets of quinine, and "Antikamnia tablets"—the latter to reduce fever and body aches.[53] The nurse distributed these at specific times, carrying a medication tray from bed to bed as she made rounds of the ward. That task was often daunting. As graduate nurse Mary C. Jones described it, "A medication list is an appalling undertaking at first: there may be thirty names on the list, some patients having as many as five or six different medications. . . . Different quantities are given—drops, drachms, ounces, and so on."[54]

Besides dispensing medications and providing patients with physical care, Ellis Island nurses were responsible for the management and appearance of the ward itself. According to one nurse, it was "the ambition of each nurse to have her ward spotlessly clean."[55] In the Ellis Island Hospital, the nurses supervised the ward maids and assistants in mopping floors and walls, changing linens, wiping down the iron beds, and sterilizing mattresses. The nurses were fortunate to have help. Earlier in the century and in other contemporaneous US hospitals, nurses themselves completed these tasks.

Preparing for and attending physician rounds was another of the nurses' responsibilities in the Ellis Island Hospital. The process was a daily ritual. First, the nurses ensured that their patients were bathed and dressed in clean gowns and covered with freshly laundered sheets prior to the physician's arrival each day. Then, the nurse accompanied the physician as he went from patient to patient, informing him of changes in the patient's vital signs, appetite, or sleep pattern; assisting him with wound dressings and other treatments; and receiving new treatment and medication orders. As one nurse described the routine, "The doctors come in to make their morning visit, the house doctor is told of any special complaints; he examines these patients . . . and leaves the new orders in my book."[56]

NURSES' ASSISTANCE IN THE BIRTH PROCESS

When a pregnant mother went into labor after landing on the island, the nurses assisted the physician with the woman's delivery. In the years before the Ellis Island Hospital had a delivery room, many of these births took place in the main hall or on the wards, the mother surrounded by portable cloth screens to ensure her privacy. In the sixty-two years during which Ellis Island functioned as an immigration station, over three hundred and fifty babies were born there.[57]

The obstetrical procedures the nurses followed were specific and based on the latest science. An 1896 article in the *Trained Nurse and Hospital Review* specified the procedures to be followed. The nurse was to bathe the mother-to-be, listen to the fetal heartbeat, and palpate the abdomen to determine the baby's position. With the onset of labor, the nurse was to put the mother to bed, "note the bearing of the patient, estimate the strength, duration and frequency of pains," and finally "determine the amount of dilatation" of the cervix. Once it was clear that delivery was imminent, the nurse scrubbed the patient's abdomen and thighs with green soap and notified the house surgeon. Having prepared a tray with "silver nitrate for the baby's eyes, chloroform, an inhaler, whiskey . . . sponges, pads, scissors, and string for the cord," the nurse then assisted the physician with the delivery, sometimes administering chloroform anesthesia under the physician's guidance. Afterwards, she cleaned the infant's mouth, weighed and bathed the baby, covered the cord with a dressing and flannel band, and then dressed the newborn in a diaper and flannel gown.[58] Since there was no nursery in the original Ellis Island Hospital, the nurse placed the baby in a wicker bassinet near the mother's bed.

In the days following the birth, the nurses continued to adhere to specific routines. For seven to ten days, the new mothers were confined to bed, during which time the nurses observed them closely for signs of uterine hemorrhage, mastitis, or postpartum fever. Providing the mother with adequate nutrition was particularly important, and for the first twenty-four hours after delivery the nurse gave her small meals of "bread and milk." Later she supplemented the mother's diet with "toast, hominy, beef broth, tea, and egg nogs," to promote her strength and ensure that her milk supply was adequate.[59]

The women delivering their babies in the Ellis Island Hospital certainly needed the extra calories and fluids. The pregnant women had sailed for weeks in the ships' steerage quarters, where they received paltry meals, often consisting of watery cabbage soup and stale bread. Combined with the inability to keep food down during episodes of nausea associated with pregnancy or rough seas, many mothers-to-be were deficient in nutrients when they arrived in New York Harbor.

NURSES ON ALERT: THE TYPHUS EPIDEMIC OF 1892

Working at the port of entry in New York Harbor, the nurses assigned to the Ellis Island Hospital had to be alert to the signs and symptoms of contagious diseases. Epidemics were frightening realities in the nineteenth century; they could "arrive suddenly, run their course, and disappear, only to return at a later date."[60] Faced with this reality, Americans often blamed the immigrants for bringing disease into the country, especially when an epidemic erupted in an overcrowded tenement district shortly after a new group of immigrants had settled there.[61]

One of the dreaded diseases of the nineteenth century was typhus, and the Ellis Island nurses' knowledge and observational skills with regard to its symptoms were put to the test just one month after the new immigration station opened. In February 1892, an epidemic of typhus fever erupted in the slums of Manhattan's Lower East Side.

The epidemic broke out soon after the arrival of the steamship *Massilia*, which carried hundreds of Jewish refugees from Russia. On January 30, 1892, the ship reached New York Harbor and made a brief inspection stop near Staten Island. In less than one hour, two physicians checked more than eight hundred passengers for signs of cholera, typhus, plague, yellow fever, or leprosy.[62] Finding "nothing medically remarkable about the bedraggled, half-starved" refugees, the health inspectors sent them on to Ellis Island, where the passengers were given another cursory screening. Only sixty-eight people were detained—not for illness but for the likelihood that they would become "a public charge" due to their economic situation.[63] Nonetheless, some of those detainees, or perhaps other passengers in first- or second-class cabins who had been sent directly to the mainland, must have been incubating typhus.

Clearly, not all cases of contagious disease could be identified aboard ship when there was still time to quarantine the patient. In fact, it was possible that an immigrant could come down with an infectious disease while they were detained on Ellis Island—even if they showed no symptoms during their initial screening. Thus, the Ellis Island nurses had to know the signs and symptoms of various infectious diseases and to be on alert for any indication of an outbreak. For typhus, nurses looked for patients experiencing "muscle pain, headache, nausea, thirst and sudden onset of an intensely high fever, along with a distinct rash and a peculiar odor.[64] Once identified, these patients were sent to one of the quarantine hospitals on nearby islands.

ELLIS ISLAND NURSES AND THE FEAR OF CHOLERA

Only seven months after the typhus epidemic on the Lower East Side, an epidemic of cholera threatened to invade Ellis Island when the "aging, slow-moving steerage steamer" *Moravia* headed into New York Harbor on August 30, 1892.[65] The lethal disease had been raging in Europe and had infected the *Moravia's* passengers, killing twenty-two people during the voyage to America. The dead had been "hastily wrapped in canvas and urgently thrown overboard—as if they were 'dead birds or garbage.'"[66] Two immigrants were acutely ill when the ship arrived.

Other ships arriving from Europe exacerbated the threat. During the month of September 1892, the *Rugia* and the *Normania* sailed into New York Harbor, bringing immigrants from Hamburg, Germany, where cholera was prevalent. On the *Rugia*, five adults traveling in steerage had died during the voyage. Another four steerage passengers were acutely ill on arrival. The situation on the *Normania* was much the same. Five deaths had occurred among steerage passengers during the voyage, as well as "a death each among first- and second-class compartments."[67] Clearly the threat of a cholera epidemic arriving in New York had to be taken seriously. Like typhus, outbreaks of cholera in the immigrant districts on the Lower East Side fueled fears that the newcomers were bringing the disease into the country.[68] According to public health officials, the health of the American public was at risk.

For the nurses on Ellis Island, protecting the health of Americans meant paying close attention to any news of an infectious disease outbreak. As was true for many other contagious diseases, a passenger might be harboring an asymptomatic cholera infection when he arrived on the island, only to develop symptoms during detention there for another reason. During shift reports in September 1892, the chief nurse no doubt reminded her staff to watch for cholera's hallmark symptoms, including "sudden cramping, vomiting, and violent diarrhea," all of which could progress rapidly to dehydration, coma, and death.[69] If a nurse identified a patient with any of these symptoms, she immediately isolated the patient and notified the physician in charge. In turn, the physician ordered the patient's transfer to one of the quarantine hospitals on nearby islands.

NURSES ASSIST EVACUATION IN THE FIRE OF 1897

The Ellis Island nurses not only provided routine hospital care and remained on alert for signs of epidemic disease, they also responded to emergencies. In 1897, when a fire broke out in the hospital, the nursing staff—by this time sufficient in size enough to allow for three nurses on night duty—did just that.

Making rounds shortly after midnight on June 15, 1897, Nurse Holz saw smoke coming from under the door leading to the immigration station. Seconds later the pine door erupted in flames and smoke billowed into the hospital, trapping more than sixty patients in their beds.[70] Coughing and yelling for help to the other night nurses, Miss Holz rushed to the children's section, grabbed up two little ones and raced for the door opening to the veranda. She had to get them to safety! Leaving them with another Ellis Island staff member, Holz raced back inside to get two other children, holding her breath for the few minutes it took to grab them and dash back outside.[71] Meanwhile, Holz's colleagues, Nurse Pfifer and a third nurse, assisted other Ellis Island employees and surgeon J. H. White in the evacuation of the remaining fifty-three patients—just before flames engulfed the hospital. Forty of the patients were adults; thirteen were children.[72] The next day, a journalist for the *Wichita Daily Eagle* reported the news from New York:

> If it was a wonder the immigrants in the main building got out all right, it was still more of a wonder that the sixty-odd patients in the hospital were saved. The nurses and doctors worked as cool and calm as any trained

firemen. They hauled the sick out on stretchers and laid them down where they would not get scorched. It was good work . . . No patients or immigrants died.[73]

Because the only telephone on the island was located in the building where the fire originated, all communication had shut down immediately and Ellis Island personnel had not been able to call for help. However, when people in Manhattan saw flames shooting up from Ellis Island, they soon realized that disaster had struck and help was needed. Fire and police patrol boats, along with "countless tugs" and "crafts of all kinds" soon surrounded the island.[74] Luckily, the ferryboat *John G. Carlisle* had docked in the Ellis Island ferry slip for the night and was available for the rescue effort.

By 1:12 a.m., with the island a "mass of flame," firemen and island personnel had loaded the patients onto the ferry and set sail to safety in Manhattan.[75] According to the *Wichita Daily News*, "When the *Carlisle* reached the Barge Office landing, ambulances from Gouverneur and Hudson Street hospitals met them. Patients were divided between the two; some later sent to Bellevue Hospital."[76]

Back on the island, the fire continued to blaze, consuming the entire wooden immigration station and other buildings in less than three hours. By morning, only three buildings remained standing—the boiler house, the coal house, and the surgeon's quarters. Everything else was "a tangle of charcoal, battered and rusted iron and ashes."[77] Among those ashes were all of the hospital records, the information contained in them lost forever.

A TEMPORARY RETURN TO THE BATTERY

For the next three years, while a new immigration station was being built on Ellis Island, steerage passengers were once again processed at the Battery. Health officers conducted inspections aboard ship or on the pier. An article in the *New York Times* on June 16, 1897, outlined the new arrangements. "Acceptable immigrants" were "passed immediately" while the sick were sent to city hospitals. Those with contagious diseases were quarantined; those detained were lodged at the barge office.[78]

The immigration arrival process changed again at the end of 1900. On December 17, 1900, a new immigration station opened on Ellis Island—this time the building was constructed with brick and limestone rather than Georgian pine. After a two-and-a-half-year hiatus, steerage-class passengers were once

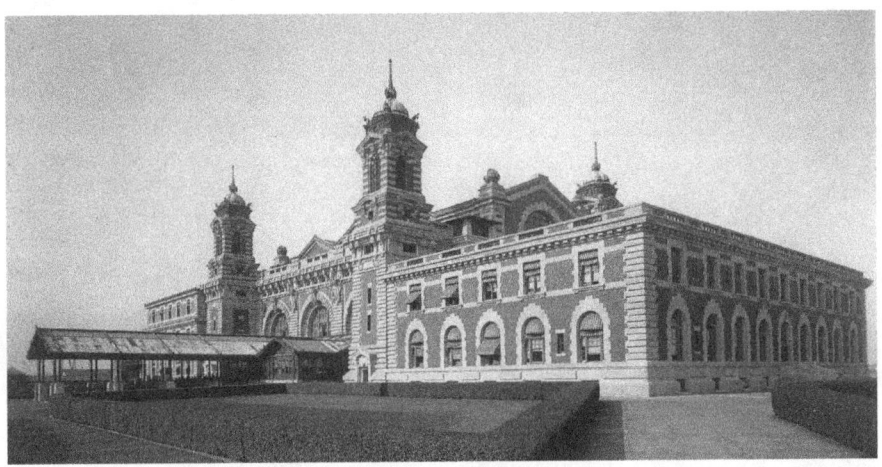

View of the Ellis Island immigration station, circa 1902–1913.
Courtesy of the Miriam and Ira D. Wallach Photography Collection, New York Public Library Digital Collections.

again ferried to the island for inspection while first- and second-class passengers received a cursory inspection on board their ships and then entered the United States directly.

In 1902, after almost a year of construction delays during which time immigrants needing medical care were sent to various city hospitals, a ninety-six-bed brick hospital was ready for occupancy on the newly constructed Island 2. The Ellis Island General Hospital was staffed by United States Public Health Service physicians—now in charge of immigration and the health of the public—and by eight nurses who had at least some formal training. One of those nurses was Margaret V. Daly, an experienced nurse who had trained at Blackwell Island Alms Hospital. Margaret began work the very same day that the General Hospital opened.[79]

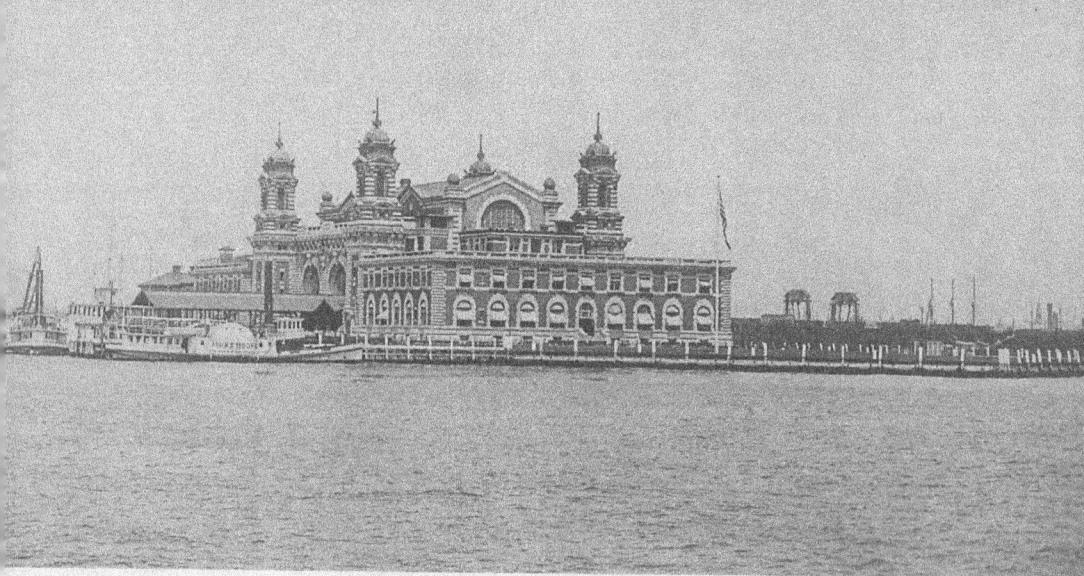

A view of Ellis Island taken from the harbor, circa 1902–1913.

Courtesy of the Miriam and Ira D. Wallach Photography Collection, New York Public Library Digital Collections.

CHAPTER 2

CARING FOR THE HUDDLED MASSES 1902–1911

I sought the appointment and after the necessary forms were filled and filed, I was accepted. . . . I reported March 1 to Dr. George W. Stoner, who was then medical officer in charge at the Station.

MARGARET V. DALY[1]

O n March 1, 1902, the new Ellis Island General Hospital building finally opened for immigrant patients, and Nurse Margaret Veronica Daly arrived for her first day of work. Simply getting there had been "quite an adventure," and Margaret felt a combination of relief and anticipation as the employee barge slowly approached the island.[2] Between her frigid predawn wait at the barge office and the icy wind whipping off the water, Margaret found the 6:20 a.m. "day force" ferry ride "not particularly appealing on a cold winter's morning."[3] It did, however, make her appreciate that nurses were required to live *and* work on Ellis Island during their employment there, eliminating the need to repeat this commute with any frequency.

The brief trip had also offered Margaret some insight into the busy day ahead. Dawn broke just minutes after the ferry departed, the golden-orange glow of sunrise slowly illuminating the Manhattan skyline and revealing a crowded New York Harbor. Rows of international steamships sat anchored just offshore; each one carried hundreds of newly arrived immigrants waiting for their own ferry ride to Ellis Island. Margaret's patients would be among them, suffering from any number of acute or chronic illnesses after spending weeks at sea in crowded and hazardous steerage conditions. These immigrants embodied the "homeless and tempest-tost [*sic*]" that Emma Lazarus had beckoned in her poem for the Statue of Liberty.[4] Caring for these "huddled masses" would present a challenge to Margaret and her fellow nurses who served in the hospital at America's "Golden Door." They would have to be prepared to care for patients with "every sort of disorder, ranging from slight injury to obscure tropical disease."[5] They would also have to abide by recently appointed Immigration Commissioner William Williams's order that the Ellis Island staff treat all immigrants with "kindness and civility."[6]

As the ferry pulled into the slip between Islands 1 and 2, Margaret gathered her wits and her two leather suitcases and set off to find the nurses' quarters. Trailing behind the other employees, she turned left off the dock toward Island 2 and carefully navigated the open-air "foot path and a narrow board bridge" connecting the main immigration center on the original island to the new hospital complex.[7] Following the procession toward the door of the new hospital building, Margaret entered the imposing three-story Georgian-style brick structure. Once inside, she followed the helpful head nods of the staff as they pointed fingers at the stairs to the second floor. She had no need to ask for directions as her starched white cap, crisp, clean uniform, and armfuls of luggage clearly identified her as one of the newly appointed nurses.

Reaching the second-floor landing, she observed other nurses rushing off to the wards, pinning on their caps and smoothing their skirts as they walked down the hallway. Not wanting to be late herself, Margaret opened the door to the nurses' dormitory and set her things in the corner of the common sitting area. She turned and stopped briefly at the threshold, moved by the views out the windows in either direction. In one direction the window across the hallway framed the Statue of Liberty in the distance. Lady Liberty stood serene, a symbolic promise of freedom and opportunity. In another direction, the view from the window in the nurses' common room showcased the grand immigration station, a symbol of the obstacles the immigrants would face before they could reach American soil.

Standing in that doorway, Margaret personified the reality of nursing on Ellis Island, which would involve navigating a professional "middle place." The General Hospital, where the nurses lived and worked, sat between the national landmark that welcomed immigrant arrivals and the building where government officials determined who was worthy of landing. The nurses stationed at Ellis Island were caught, physically and figuratively, somewhere in the

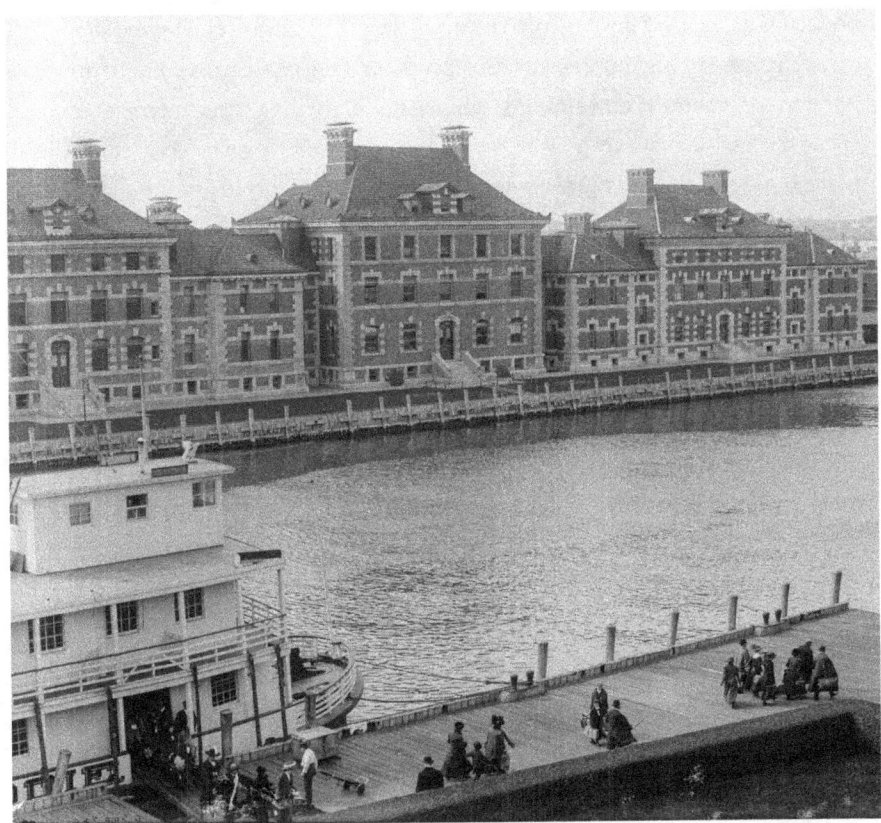

The Ellis Island General Hospital, view from the Main Building, circa 1910–1920.
Courtesy of the Library of Congress, Prints and Photographs Online Catalog.

middle—their duty to care for immigrant patients sometimes competing with their responsibility to protect the health of the American public. For Margaret, "scarcely any other field offered such an opportunity for serving God and country," and doing so would become her life's work.[8] After her arrival on that cold March day, Margaret spent the next thirty-four years nursing the sick at the Ellis Island hospitals.

NURSING AT THE ELLIS ISLAND GENERAL HOSPITAL
Returning to the first floor, Margaret entered a ward to find other nurses preparing for the arrival of their patients. Their keen eyes searched for any spots that required disinfecting, bed linens in need of straightening, or unnecessary clutter that needed organizing. Quietly surveying the room, Margaret immediately

noticed that the new hospital offered every scientific advancement and modern convenience. She also appreciated the fact that all the nurses, dressed in immaculate white uniforms and starched white caps, embodied the ideal social image of the professional nurse. As Margaret continued exploring, she began to realize that not nearly enough nurses were present to staff a hospital of this size when it reached capacity. Right now, as all ninety-six beds across the four hospital wards lay pristine and completely empty, the small team of eight nurses seemed more than adequate. However, the current absence of patients belied the actual demand for hospital care on Ellis Island, something Margaret and the rest of the staff would discover almost immediately. Nevertheless, in this moment, with sunlight streaming through the large dormer windows and glinting off disinfected marble floors, Margaret clearly realized that the design of the "general hospital for all nations" had merged the latest advances in diagnostic and therapeutic care with nursing-centered concepts about the creation of a healing environment.[9]

Finally ready after months of construction delays, the new brick and limestone Ellis Island General Hospital rivaled many of the leading institutions of the time. Hospitals in the United States had only recently evolved from charitable organizations offering mostly comfort care to the poor or destitute to highly regarded scientific institutions for the care of the sick. Those at the forefront of

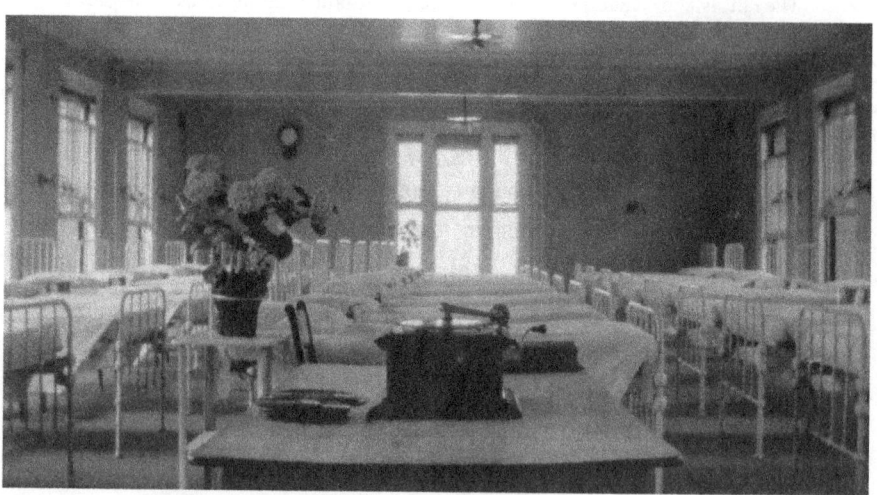

A patient ward in the Ellis Island hospitals.
Courtesy of the National Park Service, Statue of Liberty National Monument, STLI 5052.

medical progress began to embrace newer technologies like X-rays and diagnostic lab tests, designed to enhance specialized treatment for those who were acutely ill.[10] Distinguishing itself among even the most elite institutions of the era, the Ellis Island General Hospital was "modern in every respect and well equipped [with] excellent facilities for the scientific treatment of patients."[11] The building contained four separate patient wards, a central pharmacy with multiple dispensaries, a poultice room, four operating rooms, a delivery room, and a sterilizing room.[12] Additionally, the third floor of the hospital housed a branch of the Hygienic Laboratory, which would eventually become the National Institute of Health.[13]

The hospital's staff was also impressive. Both the physicians and nurses on Ellis Island were some of the most highly educated and skilled hospital personnel in the nation. Ellis Island General Hospital boasted "highly qualified medical personnel, qualified in every field of medical work—curative, preventive, and investigative."[14] All of them were United States Public Health and Marine Hospital Service physicians who had undergone a rigorous training and examination process. Formerly the Marine Hospital Service, the organization was officially renamed the USPHS in 1902 to reflect the expansion of its responsibility to include both domestic quarantine and national public health measures.[15] Complementing the elite medical staff were experienced graduate nurses hired by the USPHS to provide direct patient care. Despite the fact that they were more expensive than the student nurses who, in other hospitals, provided free labor on the wards in exchange for their education, graduate nurses undoubtedly elevated the quality of care and matched the status and high standards of the USPHS physicians. As one physician remarked, the Ellis Island hospital "was like any general hospital, except it was done with better work than the ordinary general hospital because of the number of graduate nurses."[16] Indeed, graduate nurses had the education and practical experience necessary to meet the demands they would face on Ellis Island.

In addition to their having complex scientific knowledge and expert clinical skill, Margaret and her fellow graduate nurses had adopted Florence Nightingale's environmental theory during their training. Following Nightingale's advice, the nurses espoused the idea that "to keep the sick-room in proper condition" was as important a part of the care they provided as were "more personal ministrations."[17] The USPHS physicians agreed. To that end, everything about the Ellis

Island General Hospital—from the architecture of the building and the location of appliances and treatment rooms, to the intricacies of the ward layout and available amenities—had been planned around the anticipated needs of the sick and the nurses' role in environmental management.

Following Nightingale's design for a model sick room, the wards featured high ceilings to enable optimal airflow and multiple windows on every wall to allow for adequate natural light and ventilation. Just outside the sick room was a south-facing porch, on which the patients would have ample opportunity to experience the benefits of fresh air, mild activity, and plenty of sunshine. Hygienic standards of the time also focused on the space having "as little furniture as possible, and that of the simplest kind . . . capable of being thoroughly cleaned."[18] Twelve evenly spaced iron-framed beds, each made up with crisp white linens, lined the longer walls of the rectangular-shaped wards. Between each bed stood a small table and a wooden chair. The nurses' station—a single desk at the center of the room—offered unobstructed views of the entire ward, following the recommendations in nursing textbooks that stressed, "Nothing is insignificant or beneath notice which has any bearing upon the welfare of the patient."[19]

As Margaret familiarized herself with the first-floor layout, noting the location of the dispensary, the kitchen, and the bathrooms in the long hallway between the wards, she caught a glimpse of her reflection in a window. Social standards for professional nurses insisted that she pay "the strictest attention" to her own hygiene, and in training she had been instructed that a "neat and attractive appearance" went far "toward making a nurse acceptable."[20] Relieved to see that her hair remained neatly tucked beneath her cap, Margaret briefly admired the silhouette of the USPHS uniform. She was clad in white from head to toe, her one-piece cotton dress had "a simple waist and plain sleeves . . . a four-piece skirt, from 2 to 2 ½ yards in circumference at the bottom, reaching to within 3 inches of the floor."[21] Midway between the shoulder and elbow of her left sleeve sat "a Geneva cross of maroon broadcloth," an internationally recognized symbol of neutrality that marked the nursing staff as helpers.[22] White stockings and white leather shoes completed her ensemble. Running her hands down the pearl buttons on the front of her skirt, Margaret had to admit that these uniforms both conveyed an air of clinical competence and reflected the clean and modest aesthetic of the new hospital.

Confident that she looked as professional as the other nurses, Margaret continued to explore the hospital. Focusing her attention on her surroundings rather than on herself, she didn't consider the many other characteristics she shared with the rest of the nursing staff. Chief among these characteristics were the nurses' similar demographics, which was really not surprising given the targeted application requirements for an appointment on Ellis Island. Prerequisites reflected the harsh reality of hospital nursing at the time, which challenged a woman's strength of character almost as much as the strength of her body.[23] Those interested in becoming a female "attendant" with the USPHS had to be "between the ages of 26 and 38 years, single, and graduates of a reputable training school for nurses."[24] At twenty-eight with years of diverse nursing experience and no husband or children to care for, Margaret easily fit the candidate profile. As such, she could devote herself fully to her duties on the island.

Unspoken within these rigid prerequisites was a strong racial bias, as application guidelines enabled and perpetuated systemic discrimination against

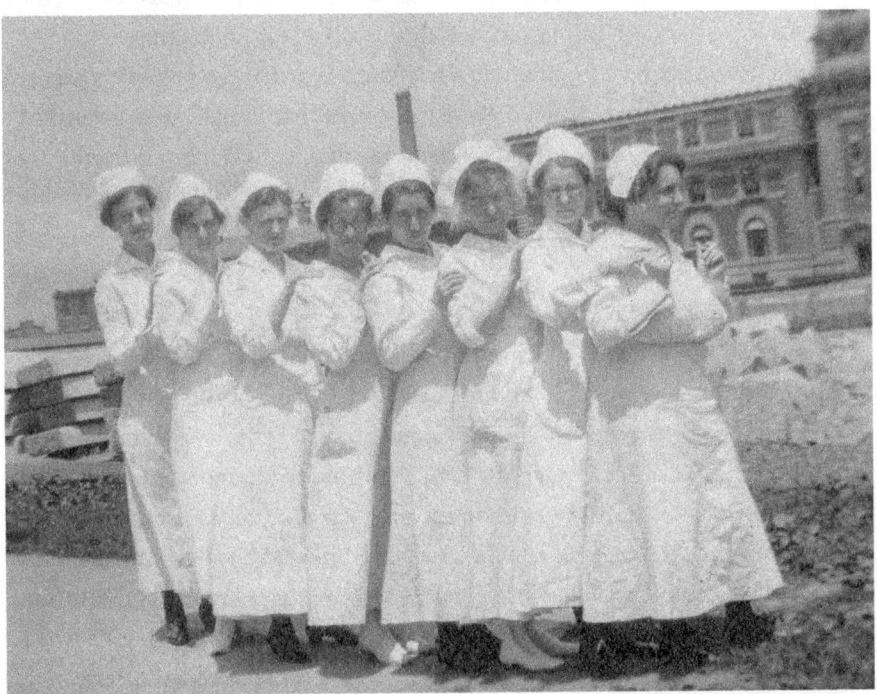

A small group of Ellis Island nurses standing outside the General Hospital.
Courtesy of the National Park Service, Statue of Liberty National Monument, STLI 5052.

hiring Black nurses. Indeed, just as they had been in the 1890s, all of the USPHS nurses on Ellis Island were White.[25] Although the application did not explicitly preclude individuals on the basis of race, it required nurses to have graduated from a "reputable" training school, thus creating a barrier for nurses of color. At the time, many national organizations, including the Red Cross Nursing Service and the Nurses Associated Alumnae, stratified nurse training programs based on the size of their affiliated hospitals or the existence of an alumni association for graduates. These requirements discriminated against students who had attended segregated schools for Blacks, the majority of which existed in smaller hospitals and lacked a recognized alumni group.[26] Intentionally or not, the constraints of the USPHS nurse application upheld the systemic racism that was pervasive throughout the nursing profession at the turn of the twentieth century.

A noisy commotion coming from the front entrance turned Margaret's attention to the fact that patients were arriving at the hospital. Young men (who she soon learned were called "runners") guided or carried the patients into the hospital's reception room.[27] Margaret realized that the runners had escorted the patients from the Main Immigration Building on Island 1 across the walkway to the hospital on Island 2. In the reception room, the patients would be officially registered and assigned to a ward. Since the patients had already been examined by the USPHS physicians in the main building and had been given a tentative diagnosis, Margaret and the other nurses in the hospital would independently initiate standard admission procedures. Her shift was about to begin.

IMMIGRANT PATIENTS

Margaret walked to the women's ward, where she had been assigned for the day, and waited for the new admissions. Hearing the voices of the patients in the receiving room, she noted their hurried and anxious tone even if she couldn't understand most of the foreign dialects. Recalling the number of steamships she had seen in the harbor earlier in the day, Margaret considered how many immigrants might soon arrive. She also reflected on what the newcomers would have already been through as they proceeded through the Great Hall in the Main Immigration Building on Island 1. Nearly all immigrants had learned that the medical exam and immigration interview on Ellis Island determined whether they would be allowed to land in the United States, but few, if any, had prepared for the possibility of a hospital stay—no wonder immigrant patients arrived at the hospital terrified and confused! They had been pulled aside by uniformed officers during the inspection and sent under guard to a separate building away from their families. Now, in addition to being ill or injured, many found themselves unable to communicate because of a language barrier. As Margaret later recalled, "They didn't want to come to the hospital because they thought it meant deportation and they could not realize that we were trying to help them."[28]

Although nurses did not participate in the medical inspection process, they soon learned about the policy-driven procedures used to sort out new arrivals. Contemporary federal laws mandated that USPHS officers examine every immigrant to identify anyone suffering from medical conditions that required mandatory exclusion and deportation. Prohibited conditions fell into one of two categories: Class A conditions, which initially specified "idiots, insane persons, [and] persons suffering from a loathsome or a dangerous contagious disease," and Class B conditions, which included any disease or defect that would increase the likelihood of a patient becoming a "public charge."[29] As USPHS physician Milton Foster understood his duties, "The medical inspection of arriving immigrants is made chiefly for two purposes: first, to see that they are strong, well, and bright enough to be able to earn a living and get along in this country; and second, to ascertain that they did not have certain diseases that they might transmit to their new neighbors in America."[30]

After the medical inspection, immigrants were required to undergo an interview with an immigration inspector, a nonmedical officer looking to identify signs of the proscribed social classes considered for mandatory exclusion: convicts, polygamists, anarchists, or any person assisted by others to come into the country. If *any* immigrant—regardless of age, nationality, or social status— was determined to have any of the medical or social exclusionary conditions, they were prohibited from entering the United States, detained at Ellis Island until someone secured return transport for them, and eventually deported to their country of origin.

By 1902 the medical inspection process on Ellis Island had been refined and standardized and typically lasted only a few hours.[31] Ferried from their steamships to the barge dock on Island 1, immigrants walked under the large, covered portico toward the entrance of the main building. There, attendants ushered everyone into separate inspection lines, men in one line, women and

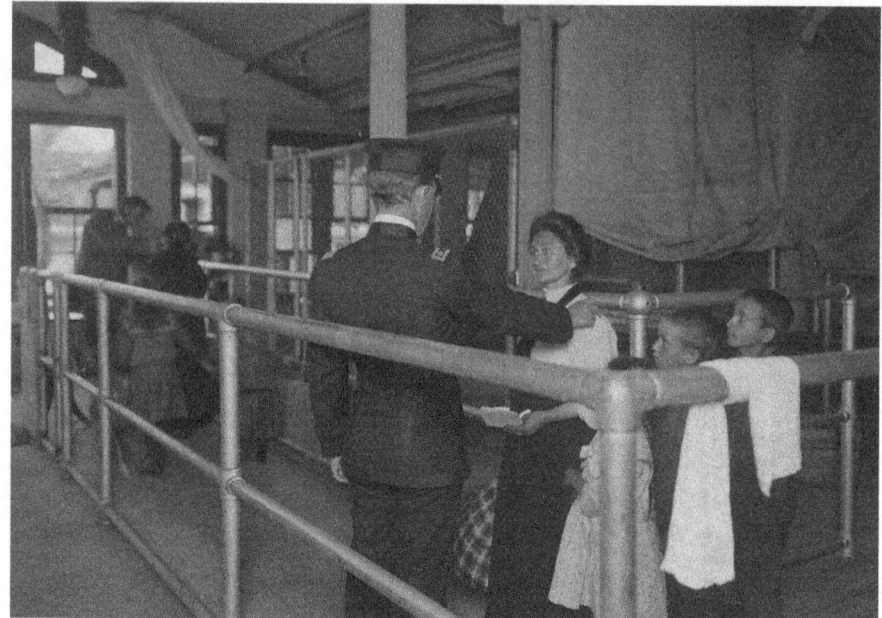

Immigrants undergoing medical examination, circa 1902–1913.
Courtesy of the Miriam and Ira D. Wallach Photography Collection, New York Public Library Digital Collections.

children in the other. Proceeding single file and carrying all their belongings, immigrants walked "the Line" toward the first USPHS inspector, who observed them from head to toe.[32] In the span of a few seconds, this physician assessed the appearance of their scalp, face, neck, hands, gait, and overall mental and physical condition. As one journalist remarked, "While the immigrant has been walking the twenty feet, the doctors have asked and answered in their own mind several hundred questions. If the immigrant reveals any intimation of disease, if he has a deformity, even down to a crooked finger, the fact is noticed."[33]

Finished with the initial inspector, immigrants continued along the Line to a second USPHS examiner, the dreaded "eye man," responsible for diagnosing visual defects or disease.[34] Facing the patient, the physician swiftly reached out with a buttonhook or his bare finger and turned out the immigrant's eyelid to allow him to adequately visualize the conjunctiva.[35] If either of the USPHS inspectors on the Line found something they felt necessitated a more thorough examination, they would write a chalk mark letter on the immigrant's lapel indicating the suspected deformity or disease. Passengers without chalk marks were immediately directed to their interview with the immigration service, while those with marks were removed from the line to undergo a more thorough "secondary inspection."[36] As USPHS physician Grover Kempf recalled, "It was a haphazard method of examination, but it was the only way it could be done" because of the sheer volume of immigrants in need of processing.[37]

After being pulled aside, immigrants with chalk marks were escorted into semiprivate assessment areas and given very detailed physical or mental exams. The USPHS physicians were instructed that "cases turned aside for special examination" should be given a "sufficiently thorough physical examination" to determine if they had "other defects besides those which primarily attracted attention."[38] Owing to the large number of immigrant arrivals at any given time, examiners tried to streamline the process by bringing those with similar chalk marks into the rooms together. Although the immigrants were separated into rooms by gender, they often suffered great distress during these exams, particularly when they were asked to undress in a room full of strangers. The experience, considered by many immigrants to be unnecessarily intrusive and culturally inappropriate, often left a lasting negative impression. As Ellis Island immigrant Emmanuel Steen candidly recalled, "I think frankly the worst memory I have of Ellis Island was the physical. . . . It's a very unpleasant memory."[39]

Depending on the results of the secondary inspection, immigrants received either an OK card or a medical detention certificate.[40] Instructions for the USPHS officers were clear: "The examiner should detain any alien or aliens as long as may be necessary to insure [*sic*] a correct diagnosis."[41] That process could include additional exams by other physicians, or any confirmatory diagnostic laboratory test. If at any point during the inspection process a USPHS physician determined that an immigrant needed acute medical care, he would send the newcomer to the Ellis Island General Hospital, "as a measure of humanity and with a view to cure."[42]

BUSY LIFE ON THE WARDS

That first day on the wards proved to be one of the busiest in Margaret's career. Since every patient was new to the hospital, Margaret completed a full admission procedure with every such individual as soon as they were assigned to her ward. Margaret made sure to meet each immigrant upon their arrival, knowing that her care began "at the first glance at a new patient."[43]

With that first glance, Margaret formed initial impressions of her patients' general condition, noticing any chalk marks on their lapel. She and the other nurses quickly learned the detailed code system utilized by the USPHS physicians during the inspection process, realizing that the markings offered insight into the patients' potential symptoms and diagnoses. Certain words—hand, nails, skin, temperature, vision, and voice—were written out in full, while other disorders were indicated with letters: *B* for back, *C*-conjunctivitis, *Ct*-trachoma, *E*-eyes, *F*-face, *Ft*-feet, *G*-goiter, *H*-heart, *K*-hernia, *L*-lameness, *N*-neck, *P*-physical and lungs, *Pg*-pregnancy, *Sc*-scalp, and *S*-senility.[44] Armed with this additional information, Margaret next assisted her patients with "an all-over bath."[45]

Experience had taught Margaret the role of therapeutic baths in quality nursing care, which could be used for cleanliness, temperature manipulation, or general relaxation. At Ellis Island General Hospital, "baths were naturally compulsory," since most immigrants had not had a proper bath for weeks during their long voyage. Nurses also needed to fully visualize the patient's skin to note color, nourishment status, any deformities or swelling and "to examine for sores" that may have been missed during the medical inspection.[46]

The bathing procedure was well-defined. The nurses escorted ambulatory patients down the hall to a common bathroom containing large porcelain tubs; for bedridden patients the nurses administered a thorough sponge bath in the bed, taking care "neither to chill nor fatigue the patient" in the process.[47] The nurses also carefully recorded itemized lists of each patient's belongings on individual tags and filed them with the reception room clerk; they sent any clothes to the laundry to be disinfected. Margaret often helped place her patient's "petticoats and socks and shoes" in "a large burlap bag" and sent it to the laundry facilities in the hospital outbuilding next door.[48]

When she completed her patients' baths, Margaret dressed them in white cotton hospital gowns, helped them get comfortable in bed, and began to vigilantly observe their vital signs and physical condition. She carefully made these assessments, noting the frequency, rhythm, and force of every patient's pulse; the rate, depth, and regularity of their respirations; and the temperature and degree of moisture to their skin.[49] Margaret also observed her patients' expression for signs of pain and assessed their level of attentiveness and engagement, an interesting challenge since few patients spoke English. She recorded the vital signs in the patient charts at the nurses' station and took mental note of her observations to share with the doctor during physician rounds. Should her patient display abnormal symptoms or have vital signs well outside the expected range, Margaret knew to immediately notify the senior ward nurse, who would then contact the supervising USPHS physician for further instructions. When she had made her stable patients comfortable, Margaret continued to observe for any changes in their condition, taking their vital signs at specific intervals.

Once per shift, the supervising physician checked on all the patients and asked nurses for concise, objective accounts of the clinical situation. Margaret's ability "to observe accurately, and to describe intelligently," a patient's condition distinguished her as a trained nurse.[50] After the USPHS physician wrote orders for additional diagnostic tests, medicines, diet, and therapeutic treatments for every patient on the ward, the nurses were responsible for carrying out all those orders in a timely manner. Like the other graduate nurses on Ellis Island, Margaret's nursing training and varied work experience prepared her well for success in the General Hospital. She immediately fulfilled a physician's directives; for patients who needed additional diagnostic tests, Margaret collected urine and sputum specimens for routine cultures and assisted those who needed X-rays. In the dispensary located between the wards, Margaret prepared common drugs she had learned about in the latest *Materia Medica* for nurses, administering them to her patients according to the prescribed quantity, route, and frequency.[51] For patients with inflammation, Margaret headed to the poultice room, where she mixed linseed, oatmeal, charcoal, or bread meal with boiling water and placed the mixture on strips of muslin to make a poultice. These therapeutic poultices supplied warmth to the affected area, softened the patient's tissues, and relieved their tension. Sometimes she sprinkled laudanum over the poultices to relieve her patient's pain.[52] Margaret also carefully disinfected and bandaged any wounds and applied wooden splints or plaster bandages to patients with fractures.

Immigrant patients were frequently admitted to the hospital due to pneumonia. With a first glance, Margaret easily recognized the signs of the

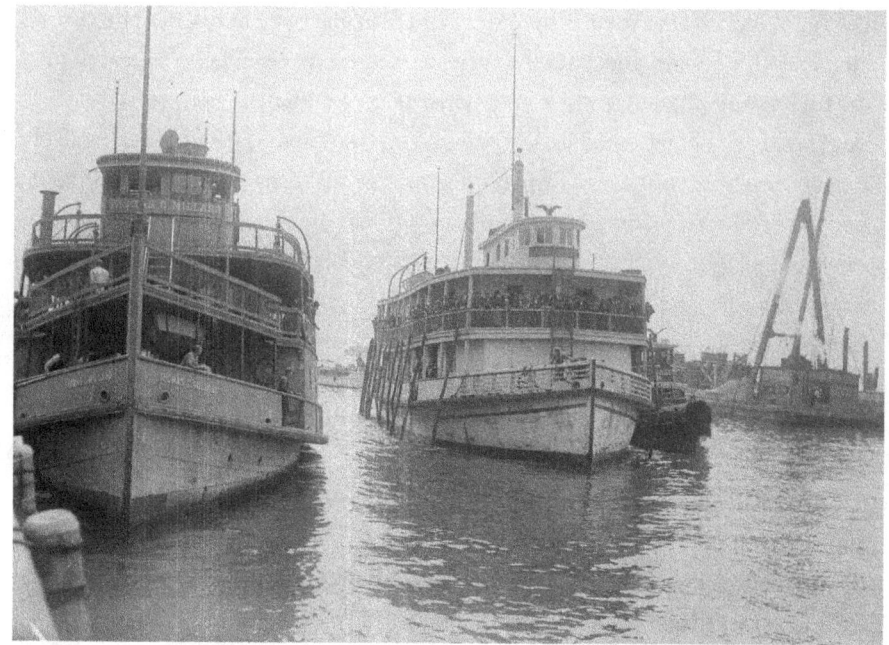

Immigrant barges at Ellis Island, 1920.
Courtesy of the Library of Congress, Prints and Photographs Online Catalog.

infection: flushed cheeks, labored breathing, and a painful, productive cough. She immediately escorted these patients to bed, knowing they "should be kept perfectly quiet, being permitted no conversation or exertion that may agitate or excite to effort."[53] After giving her patients a gentle but thorough bed bath, Margaret carefully assessed them and recorded their vital signs, paying particular attention to each patient's temperature, pulse, and respirations. She spent time just watching them breathe, noting how her patients positioned themselves, whether their nostrils flared, and if they had to use extra muscles in their chests to get enough oxygen. If she noticed a dusky skin tone, blue lips, and quick, shallow breaths indicating serious complications, Margaret alerted the physician on call.

Prior to the discovery of antibiotics, treatment for pneumonia was "directed principally toward making the patient comfortable."[54] Nurses treated the pain and inflammation of the chest with topical applications, alternating hot poultices, cold packs, and ice compresses. Margaret did the same. She also ensured her pneumonia patients received plenty of fresh air; she bundled them up and sat them beside an open window or brought them outside for sunlight therapy and fresh breezes off the harbor.

Despite the recent scientific and technological advances in medicine, nursing care at the turn of the twentieth century remained largely supportive. As was true with the treatment for pneumonia, much of the nurses' work on Ellis Island still involved everyday domestic tasks and emotional support. Margaret was responsible for feeding and bathing her patients, as well as assisting them out of bed for toileting or mild exercise. Beds had to be clean and fresh at all times, so the nurses removed any soiled linen and replaced it to prevent their patients' any discomfort. Since she also needed to ensure the ward environment remained comfortable, Margaret frequently opened and closed windows to maintain proper temperature and ventilation.

As the day wore on, Margaret realized that the constant stream of new patients never slowed. Just as she finished settling her latest admission, Margaret had barely enough time to check on the others in the rest of the ward before someone called her to help admit the next patient. Glancing out the window as she walked the long hallway back to the reception room, Margaret watched yet another barge full of immigrant arrivals dock outside the Main Immigration Building. Although she knew the day shift technically ended at 6:00 p.m., she expected to stay on duty until all passengers from the last steamship had been processed, just in case an immigrant needed to be hospitalized.[55] Later that night, after she had reported to the overnight attendant and slowly trudged upstairs to her room, Margaret realized that the on-island living arrangements would be as much a necessity as a convenience.

THE SCHEDULE AND STRUCTURE OF NURSING WORK

Days and weeks passed in much the same manner as had her first day, and it soon became clear to Margaret that long and hectic shifts would be the norm rather than the anomaly on Ellis Island. Though the work at the hospital "was quite arduous," Margaret later recorded that "the years flew past."[56] The annual number of patients admitted to the General Hospital increased exponentially as the number of immigrants increased; after treating 913 patients in 1902, Ellis Island nurses encountered an average of nearly 7,000 patients every year until 1916.[57] With only eight nurses on staff in the early years, Margaret and the other nurses were pushed to their physical and emotional limits. Indeed, it was "not difficult to imagine the difficulties this small number had to contend with."[58] The nurses' shifts lasted "practically all day and often late into the night," and each nurse received only a half day off each week "provided [they] could be spared."[59] During one particularly grueling stretch, Margaret "worked steadily for six weeks at a time without a single day off."[60] To succeed in such a challenging work environment, Margaret and the other nurses leaned on one another and on a rigid hierarchy that organized the nurses within the hospital.

Given the demanding nature of hospital work at the time, the USPHS adopted a strict chain of command that nurses followed to ensure swift, efficient work and organized collective action. That chain of command also aligned with the military-style rank system that classified medical officers of the USPHS. A familiar structure that Margaret and her fellow nurses had internalized from their days as trainees in nursing school, the hierarchy determined each nurse's specific duties and their level of individual accountability on the wards.[61] Staff nurses were overseen by senior ward nurses and a chief nurse, who operated "under the immediate orders of the medical officer in charge of the hospital" and took responsibility for all nursing activities on the island.[62]

In addition to clarifying individual responsibilities and promoting efficiency on busy wards, nursing leaders embraced the military hierarchy as a method of legitimizing their profession in the male-dominated medical sphere. To elevate the status of their profession, nurses carefully negotiated long-standing social and professional gender norms. They gained acceptance and legitimacy in the hospital when they not only adhered to rigid morality and dress codes but also maintained complete subordination to physicians. Since the start of nurse training school, Margaret had learned that nursing "is not and cannot be democratic . . . to this end complete subordination of the individual nurse to the work as a whole is as necessary for her as for the soldier."[63] So long as nurses upheld absolute fidelity to physicians and proved themselves through the quality of their work, their profession could find a respected place within the hospital. As historian Patricia D'Antonio notes, "Nurses welcomed the military analogies because they referred not only to the male medical head but also to their own legitimate power to search for relevant pieces of medical data, to negotiate new meanings about a particular patient's symptoms, and to create new ideas about the significance of a particular clinical situation."[64]

Margaret's skill and dedication on the wards quickly caught the eye of the supervising USPHS physicians, and in 1906 she was promoted to chief nurse, a position she would hold until her retirement in 1936. Chief Medical Officer W. C. Billings described Margaret as "without the shadow of a doubt the best qualified nurse" for the chief position.[65] The title involved a great deal of responsibility, both clinical and administrative.

In addition to supervising the quality and completion of all nursing work throughout the Ellis Island General Hospital, Chief Nurse Margaret inspected every ward, the operating room, and the nurses' quarters on a daily basis.[66] As an administrator she made daily ward assignments, approved individual nurse schedules, wrote monthly reports, and handled all disciplinary procedures. Margaret was also responsible for maintaining the morale of all nurses, ward maids, and female attendants in the hospital, the number of which grew to more than thirty by 1913.[67] Her colleagues found her to be particularly well-suited for the position, citing a "very unusual ability to handle her nurses and get from them the best work of which they [were] capable."[68]

A CHALLENGING ENVIRONMENT OF CARE

Although Margaret had come to Ellis Island with years of varied nursing experience at multiple hospitals in New York state, nothing could have prepared her for the distinctive challenges she faced working for such a "complex organization."[69] Beyond the logistical idiosyncrasies and environmental limitations inherent in operating a hospital on a man-made island in the middle of a busy harbor each day, the nurses of Ellis Island had to cope with a broad range of patient diagnoses, language barriers, cultural differences, limited patient beds, and a lack of specialty facilities. As chief nurse, Margaret also had to manage nurse staffing and scheduling without being able to accurately predict the number of daily admissions or how long any patient might need hospitalization. USPHS physician Milton H. Foster summed it up as follows:

> The hospital facilities at Ellis Island must be sufficient to handle any epidemic or other disaster which might happen in a good-sized community. It is by no means unusual to receive one hundred cases or more at the hospital in one day. The task of admitting, examining, treating, and housing this number of new patients in five or six hours, would tax the capacity of the largest hospitals in the country.

Here the problem is also complicated by the fact that practically
none of the patients speak English. Furthermore, an approximately
equal number must be discharged, if possible, to make room for the
newcomers.[70]

Margaret admitted that these additional challenges "made the work of the
hospital very heavy," particularly for nurses. As the most frequent point of
contact for patients, in addition to being tasked with maintaining cleanliness
and order on the wards, nurses learned to moderate their own expectations
and develop creative solutions to help their patients as best as they could. Over
time, and often through trial and error, Margaret became "particularly proficient in the care of immigrants and in understanding of the problems and
needs" of this specific group of patients.[71]

The immigrants who arrived on Ellis Island had traveled "literally from
the farthest corners of the earth," spending weeks crossing the Atlantic Ocean
in crowded steerage conditions.[72] Therefore, the hospital nurses needed to be
ready to address every possible diagnosis, from obscure tropical diseases to
common, everyday ailments. The wards in the General Hospital were divided
only by gender; consequently, on every shift, the nurses cared for patients of
all ages and cultures with an astoundingly wide range of illnesses and injuries.
Even for someone like Margaret, who came to the island with experience in general nursing, obstetric and pediatric care, and contagious disease nursing, the
sheer breadth and depth of knowledge required to adequately serve her patients
proved challenging.[73] Besides caring for their patients' physical needs, Ellis
Island nurses also grappled with how best to meet the unique emotional and
social demands of sick immigrants who were new to the country, its customs,
and its language, all while adhering to the strict USPHS procedures. As Margaret recalled, "I have had to understand the viewpoint and language of every
nationality and respect it and at the same time abide by rules."[74]

Basic communication was the most challenging aspect of the nurses' work,
however. Only a small percentage of their patients spoke English, and for years
interpreters were not employed exclusively for hospital services. By 1911, interpreters on Ellis Island were at least "slightly acquainted" with thirty-six different languages, but successful communication depended entirely upon which
interpreters were currently scheduled, what languages those interpreters were

familiar with, and what languages or dialects were spoken by the immigrants.[75] As Immigration Commissioner William Williams described, "Our interpreters cope with the situation as best they can, and that means in some instances that they cannot cope with it."[76] According to Dr. Milton Foster, all hospital staff had "picked up a few useful words in several tongues" and an interpreter could be borrowed only when it became "absolutely necessary."[77]

In order to explain everything from hospital protocols and specialized treatments to diet choices and visiting hours, Margaret usually turned to more primitive methods of communication. When executed well, her head nods, funny faces, and finger pointing proved remarkably effective. Although she admitted to learning "a smattering of all languages and dialects," Margaret truly believed that "the universal language is pantomime. If I used my hands everyone seemed to understand."[78] Her patients agreed, particularly the younger ones. Hospitalized on Ellis Island at the age of six, John Henry Wilberding recalled that he and his brother "couldn't understand what they were talking about. But they had sign language, and we did everything in sign language. And I don't know how it worked but it worked beautifully."[79]

Unfortunately, misunderstandings between nurses and patients on Ellis Island frequently extended beyond a simple language barrier. Many immigrant families came from rural areas and had never seen a hospital or many of the instruments, like thermometers or bedpans, that nurses utilized to provide care; even everyday items like iron beds, showers, and toilets were new experiences for some immigrants. Margaret remembered the shock of finding several of her patients sleeping on the floor underneath a fresh and clean bed simply because they had never seen one before.[80] Even the nurses themselves were novelties. As one former patient recalled, "I remember that it was so strange, you know. I'd never seen a nurse before in my life . . . she's just straightening her beds up, and kind of making things right."[81]

Margaret also discovered that adequately feeding immigrant patients at Ellis Island hospital proved especially challenging since they had distinctive cultural preferences and had limited exposure to traditional American foods. The ward maids provided the patients with three meals a day, but the food was "so different from that of most countries" that ensuring a proper diet was always "a source of great struggle."[82] Ward maid Josephine Friedman concurred, saying "they couldn't get used to our food . . . it was so different from what they were used to."[83] Patients frequently turned down the food that was offered, with one exception. As Josephine recalled, "Every one of them liked potatoes. You couldn't give them enough potatoes." Because of this, Margaret found that "giving the nourishing well-balanced meals really was a problem."[84]

In addition to patient-specific challenges, Ellis Island nurses faced difficulties directly related to the hospital itself. Even prior to the opening of the new building in 1902, officials worried about the hospital's limited bed capacity amid the rising number of immigrants, asserting that "the new immigrant hospital . . . will not afford sufficient ward space for the service."[85] Those fears soon proved justified. Margaret deemed the original ninety-six-bed hospital "inadequate to take care of the large number of sick immigrants," and because the volume of patients frequently exceeded capacity, "it was always necessary to crowd in additional cots to provide for the overflow."[86] Out of necessity to alleviate overcrowding, officials maintained contracts with local area hospitals, particularly Long Island College Hospital, for many years. Commissioner Williams found the arrangement "utterly inadequate," and a 1903 presidential commission concluded that "this lack of space has been injurious to all concerned."[87]

In response, Congress appropriated funds for two new additions to the Ellis Island General Hospital on Island 2. Margaret recalled that in 1905—only three years after the new hospital building had opened—"a new wing was built, adding about fifty beds to the hospital capacity," but even that increase proved "far from adequate."[88] Another addition, "almost double the size" of the original general hospital building, was finally completed in June 1910.[89] Margaret found the new building, which consisted of "four wards, bringing the total capacity up to 267," quite an improvement from when she first arrived on the island.[90]

HANDLING CONTAGIOUS CASES

Despite the increased bed capacity in the General Hospital, Ellis Island still lacked the appropriate space and resources to treat immigrants diagnosed with a contagious illness. This significant vulnerability had worried and frustrated the USPHS nurses and physicians since the island was first established in 1892. Although New York State officials searched every international steamship for "all diseases of a quarantinable nature, including cholera, smallpox, and yellow fever," they could not identify all contagious cases during their initial, often cursory, inspection.[91] As a result, immigrants suffering from more common communicable diseases like measles and scarlet fever frequently landed on Ellis Island in need of immediate medical attention. Without a "suitable building" in which to isolate contagious individuals on Island 2, it was "not possible to properly care for them," so the USPHS established agreements with the New York City Health Department and other local hospitals to transfer these patients as soon as they were identified.[92] Within a few months of her arrival on Ellis Island, Margaret determined that this was "an expensive and inconvenient procedure," creating an excessive burden not only for immigrant patients but also for the USPHS personnel and the immigration officials.[93]

For sick immigrants, the complex transfer process and subsequent hospital stay often proved deadly. Prior to the introduction of antibiotics and reliable vaccines, diphtheria, measles, scarlet fever, and whooping cough posed a serious health threat to everyone, particularly children. In 1910 these "contagious diseases of childhood" accounted for more than 30 percent of all deaths in US children aged five to nine years.[94] Treatment at the time was largely supportive, and individual outcomes often rested on the patient's prior health status and the timing and quality of nursing care they received. Without a contagious disease facility on the island where nurses could provide care immediately, immigrant patients were at a distinct disadvantage. Steerage class passengers usually came from rural and/or poor areas and often began their immigration journey in poor health, further increasing their vulnerability to illness.[95] The crowded steerage conditions onboard the ship also served as "a propagating bed for disease," and steamships often arrived at Ellis Island "with a large number of children already sick and helpless."[96] By the time the USPHS officers recognized that passengers needed treatment, they subjected the ailing patients to exposure to the elements through a tedious ambulance transfer process from the island to any one of the contracted hospitals scattered across the city, where the quality of care varied widely. These patients, most of them children, suffered mortality rates that were deemed "nigh appalling."[97]

Maintaining contracts with mainland hospitals also proved costly and logistically problematic for the USPHS. During the 1906 fiscal year alone, more than twenty-five hundred immigrant patients were transported to outside hospitals by ambulance. These admissions required more than fifty thousand treatment days among multiple hospitals and cost more than $100,000.[98] Although a federal law required that steamship companies pay the cost of acute medical care for any immigrant passengers who were admitted to the Ellis Island General Hospital, the billing process for care received at contracted hospital facilities proved much more complex. Additionally, immigration officials lamented the difficulty in keeping track of medically detained immigrants in hospitals scattered across New York City, where they were "beyond the immediate supervision of the Government."[99]

The immigration officials lobbied in earnest for a suitable "contagious" facility to be built on a new section of Ellis Island, and Congress began appropriating funds for such a building in March 1903. Unfortunately, the Contagious Disease Hospital would not be ready for patients until June 1911, the process hindered by piecemeal congressional funding and the complexities of developing such a facility. Before construction crews could build a medical complex that would ensure "freedom from danger of contagion according to modern ideas of hospital construction," they first had to create an entirely new island on which to place the hospital.[100]

In spring 1905 construction teams began staking the large, rectangular outline of Island 3, located just a few hundred feet off the southern coast of Island 2 toward Liberty Island. Watching from the General Hospital, Margaret and the rest of the nurses realized with some disappointment that their favorite swimming area had just become a construction zone.[101] Over the next year, barges carrying excess dirt and debris from the excavation of the New York City subway tunnels gradually filled in the space, until the nearly five-acre island emerged.[102] Construction of the Contagious Disease Hospital began soon after.

Watching the new complex take shape, Margaret noticed the differences between the two Ellis Island hospitals. Rather than a single large building like the General Hospital, the contagious disease facility featured several smaller pavilions connected by an open central corridor spanning the length of Island 3. Projecting out from both sides of the long walkway, the plain rectangular buildings were evenly spaced and staggered to prevent any cross ventilation. In fact, each one could be "separately administered and quarantined" in the event of an unexpected outbreak.[103] Margaret also appreciated the numerous large windows on every floor because she knew that "an abundant supply of sunlight is absolutely essential, and the ventilation must be continuous" in the treatment of contagious illness.[104] In addition to patient pavilions, the contagious disease complex included a three-story central administrative building containing the nurses' quarters, staff dining rooms, and operating room. At one end of the complex was a separate kitchen, the powerhouse and laundry facility, and a morgue with autopsy amphitheater. At the other end was a medical staff house.[105] Though completed in 1909, the cost of the hospital complex had exceeded congressional funding, leaving no budget to purchase medical equipment, furnishings, or general supplies. Two more years passed before the hospital was fully operational.

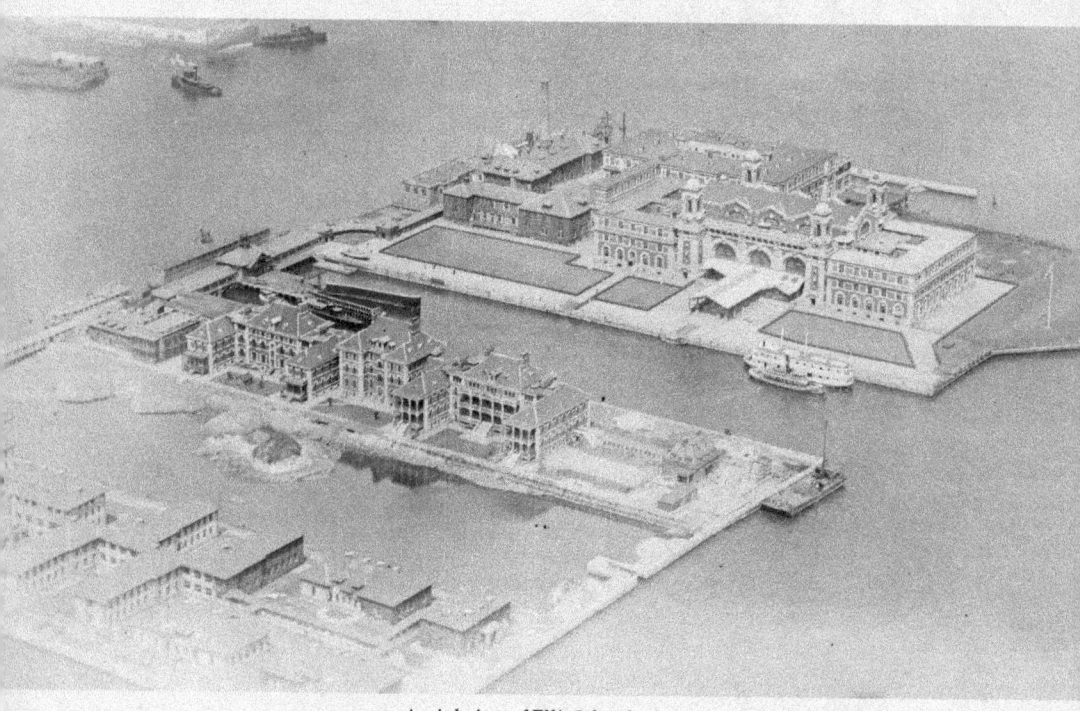

Aerial view of Ellis Island, circa 1915–1920.
Courtesy of the Library of Congress, Prints and Photographs Online Catalog.

CHAPTER 3

NURSING CARE IN THE CONTAGIOUS DISEASE HOSPITAL 1911–1917

In 1911 a new island, built by fill-ins, reared itself above the tide,
and a complete contagious hospital of about 380 beds was
erected on the site and opened for service.

MARGARET V. DALY[1]

On June 18, 1911, two days before the sprawling Contagious Disease Hospital officially opened, Margaret Daly toured the buildings on Island 3, mentally reviewing her weekly assignments while inspecting the wards to ensure they were ready to receive patients. She had recently made a habit of coming here on Sundays after taking the ferry to and from Mass at Our Lady of the Rosary Parish on the Battery. She always delighted in the solitude and fresh air as she walked up and down the long, open corridor between the empty buildings.[2] Unlike previous Sundays, however, the energy on the island today was palpable; a flurry of activity surrounded her as staff moved in, checked patient rooms and equipment, and stocked and prepped the diet kitchen. As the highest-ranking nurse on Ellis Island, Margaret managed all these tasks while temporarily acting as chief nurse of both the General Hospital and the Contagious Disease Hospital. She recognized that her new assignment would more than double her workload, but she also knew the Contagious Disease Hospital "was definitely a step forward" for the immigrant patients she served.[3] Ready for the challenge, Margaret set out to assess the rest of the buildings and check in with the nurses who had arrived. Right now, she had plenty of work to do. She did, however, look forward to the time when another chief nurse would be hired specifically for the Contagious Disease Hospital.

Surveying the exterior of the new medical complex, Margaret applauded its practicality, despite its utilitarian aesthetic. Every detail of the buildings on Island 3 had been selected to minimize the risk of disease spread, including the fact that each ward was isolated from the next. All nursing procedures had fittingly followed suit. Meticulous protocols had been developed for everything from patient transport and visitation policies to the method and frequency of sterilization for linens, instruments, and patient rooms.[4] The graduate nurses appointed to the Contagious Disease Hospital had come to Ellis Island with training and ward experience in the care of patients with "germ diseases," but Margaret knew that all staff members—including the ward maids, attendants, cooks, and laundresses—needed explicit instructions on the basic principles of disease transmission and how to apply them to their professional duties.[5] On Island 3, no responsibility was "of greater gravity than the prevention of infection."[6]

Recognizing that even the best intelligent building design could not overcome any careless practices, Margaret knew she had to set clear and stern expectations with the staff for them to adhere to protocols and establish a strict hierarchy of accountability. All staff members needed instructions on their role in infection prevention and to be taught how to protect themselves and others while working with the contagious patients. That training would have to emphasize that "infectious diseases are taken and carried by contact."[7] As such, Margaret would demonstrate proper hand washing, show the correct method of donning gowns, gloves, and caps before entering a patient's room, and explain the USPHS rules for the sterilization of the patient's items—even the mattresses needed to be sterilized in the oversized autoclave housed on the island.[8]

Margaret had to establish a strict hierarchy of accountability among her staff. They needed to follow infection prevention techniques "without ever making exceptions" because any mistake or breach in protocol "might prove disastrous."[9] She also planned to meet privately with the head nurse of each ward, imploring them to "watch vigilantly for any violation" in procedure and redirect or retrain their staff as necessary.[10]

Two days later, as the nurses in the Contagious Disease Hospital began to admit patients, they and the ward maids witnessed how the building design and the infection prevention guidelines worked in harmony to reduce the spread of illness. Although the hospital initially was built to serve immigrant patients with confirmed contagious diseases who had fallen ill aboard the steamships, the nurses soon admitted immigrants who had developed symptoms of contagious illness while being treated in the General Hospital or while waiting in the detention areas on Island 1.[11]

NURSING CARE OF CONTAGIOUS CASES

The protocols were clear. Whenever a USPHS physician identified a potential contagious case, the nurses called the administrative building on Island 3 and requested a hand ambulance and an attendant to transport the patient. A male attendant, clad in a long white isolation gown, brought the sterilized ambulance cart to pick up the patient and delivered them to a small waiting area on the west end of the contagious disease complex near the isolation wards. The hand ambulance—a pushcart with a removable prairie schooner top—accomplished two very important goals: it kept the patient isolated to shield others from contamination and protected the patient from exposure to the elements during the 150 to 300 yard transport from the other islands "through passageways and over bridges exposed to the open air."[12] Once the patient reached the waiting area, the

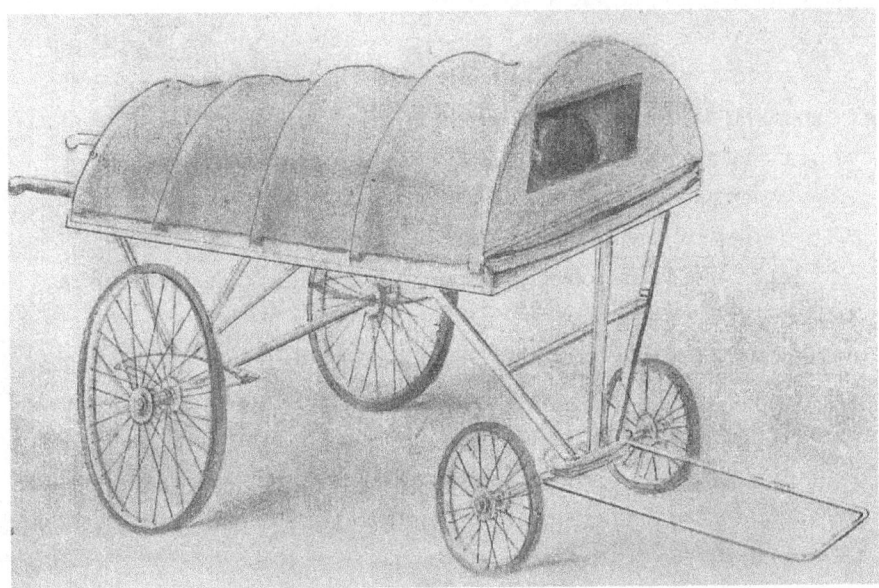

Illustration of hand ambulance used on Ellis Island, 1918.
Courtesy of the Treasury Department, United States Public Health Service.

admitting physician on Island 3 assigned them to a specific isolation ward and instructed the attendant to bring them there. The officer then telephoned the head nurse and alerted her to the new admission.

Much of the nurses' work in admitting and caring for a contagious patient mirrored the procedures in the General Hospital. In the Contagious Disease Hospital, however, all nursing activities, including feeding, bathing, toileting, administering medications, and checking vital signs, were performed while the nurses wore protective clothing. At least three long-sleeved gowns, caps, and pairs of rubber gloves hung on hooks outside the entrance of every patient room, one each for the doctor, nurse, and ward maid. Attendants resupplied the hooks with fresh, clean gowns daily. Alongside the protective clothing sat a basin of 2 percent creolin solution so the staff could immediately sterilize their hands and other items upon entering or exiting the ward.[13] Any individual who entered the Contagious Disease Hospital was expected to be fully gowned, with their cap "properly drawn and the buttons fastened."[14] Instructions were also clear regarding the proper removal of the protective clothing: "Under no circumstances" was a person to "parade in the corridors or go from one cubicle to another or go from a ward into a corridor until the gown" had "been removed."[15] The nursing staff came to appreciate the stringent and exacting methods of instruction they received in infection prevention. Having been "thoroughly trained in the proper technique of the place," the nurses allowed the elaborate protocols to become a second nature to them. This acceptance proved to be very useful given that hospital operations seemed to change constantly.[16]

How the individual wards were laid out was another key difference between the two hospitals. The traditional open ward design found in the General Hospital ran counter to the goal of preventing the spread of highly communicable illnesses. Isolation wards in the Contagious Disease Hospital were therefore broken down into twelve smaller observation units, six rooms in a row on each side of a common hallway. Partitions between each unit contained a large glass window, and the patients' beds were placed near or in front of the window. This allowed nurses to see every patient on their ward at all times, while also providing isolated children the opportunity to safely interact with others in the adjoining units—albeit through a window.[17] Each room was equipped with running hot and cold water. To prevent physicians and nurses from using the same instruments among patients, the staff supplied each room with its own

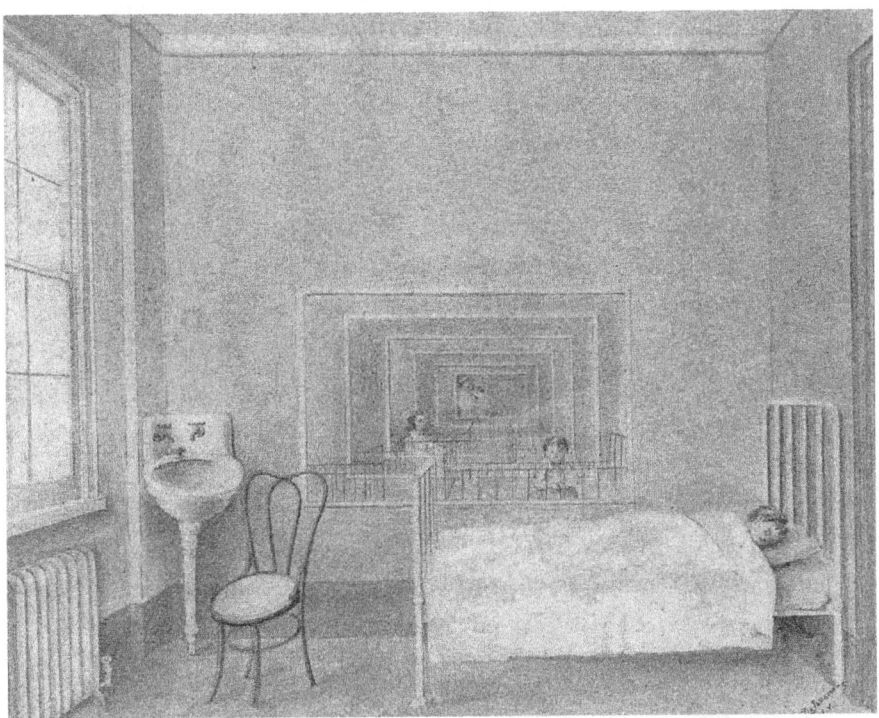

Illustration of small isolation unit in the Contagious Disease Hospital on Ellis Island, 1918.
Courtesy of the Treasury Department, United States Public Health Service.

equipment, which included a drop-light attachment for examining a patient's ears and throat and a clinical thermometer.

Patients remained in the smaller isolation units until they had completed a specified period of observation and quarantine and the supervising physician had confirmed a diagnosis. From there, patients were transferred to one of the disease-specific convalescent wards for further treatment. These wards more closely resembled those found in the General Hospital, except for the fact that patients were separated by diagnosis *and* gender. The patients remained hospitalized until they had fully recovered from their illness and from any complications they had suffered. Their bed was then available for a new admission.

In the Contagious Disease Hospital, the seasonal timing of admissions fluctuated considerably. In some months of the year the nurses on Island 3 cared for only a handful of immigrant patients. The volume of admissions also varied on any given day. Periodically, "with less than an hour's warning more than fifty patients" arrived, "suffering from different contagious diseases."[18]

Other seemingly constant changes to hospital operations also affected admissions. Sometimes the USPHS physicians modified the admission criteria, which changed the types of patients the nurses treated on the wards. In 1912 only patients with confirmed cases of contagious illnesses like measles, diphtheria, meningitis, chicken pox, whooping cough, and scarlet fever were sent to the Contagious Disease Hospital on Island 3, but physicians soon sent over patients with favus, trachoma, ringworm, and hookworm as well. Each additional disease diagnosis meant that the staff had to adjust the placement and design of the wards.[19] As USPHS assistant surgeon J. G. Wilson described, the Contagious Disease Hospital was constantly "in the process of making, large wards being divided into smaller, and interior alterations being made in order to evolve gradually a more perfect system."[20] Meticulous nursing care was undoubtedly a crucial component of that system. By 1916 that kind of perfect care had helped to drastically reduce the incidence of cross infection and the overall mortality rate in the Contagious Disease Hospital.[21] One of the greatest improvements in the survival rate occurred in patients with measles.

MEASLES ON ELLIS ISLAND

Before the Contagious Disease Hospital even opened its doors, USPHS physicians anticipated the need to treat numerous young patients suffering from measles. While planning the building design and layout, Ellis Island's long-standing chief medical officer George W. Stoner reported that measles constituted "more than 85% of the cases of contagious diseases" identified among immigrant arrivals and that "the provision for separate buildings and for each ward as an administrative unit" was "very important."[22] When the hospital complex was finally completed, it included eight separate pavilions, each housing two wards designated solely for the treatment of measles cases. The USPHS certainly needed the dedicated space; over the next few years, more than twenty-six hundred patients diagnosed with measles were admitted to the Contagious Disease Hospital. In fact, according to a 1918 report, measles cases accounted for more than 60 percent of all admissions.[23]

One of the most contagious of all known diseases in the early twentieth century, measles was known to spread "with pandemic ferocity" among children and others who had no previous exposure to the illness.[24] Crowded conditions in the steerage compartments of international steamships only exacerbated the problem. USPHS surgeon Milton H. Foster, who worked on Ellis Island in 1915, remembered one instance in which "94 cases of measles were taken from the steerage compartment of one vessel."[25] Despite being a leading cause of death and serious complications in the early twentieth century, measles was "considered relatively harmless by the great majority," likely because of its common and pervasive occurrence. At the time, overall mortality rates for measles varied between 1 and 6 percent but were largely dependent on age and overall health, with extremely high case fatality rates observed among infants and toddlers.[26] Between 1912 and 1916, in the Contagious Disease Hospital more than 70 percent of all deaths from measles occurred in patients under the age of four.[27]

The unique circumstances surrounding immigrant patients on Ellis Island made measles outbreaks even more problematic. As USPHS assistant surgeon J. G. Wilson described,

> It is impossible to imagine any more unfavorable conditions for recovery
> from measles than to be taken sick in the steerage in transit to the
> United States, and then, either in the height of the disease or before
> convalescence is well established, to be transported in overcrowded
> barges from the New York City docks to the immigrant station at
> Ellis Island. Besides the unfavorable sanitary conditions necessarily
> surrounding this procedure, the patient has almost invariably been
> exposed to the risk of cross infection before he reaches the hospital.[28]

Indeed, mortality rates for measles in the Contagious Disease Hospital remained particularly high when an outbreak occurred during the transatlantic voyage. By the time immigrant passengers arrived at Ellis Island, dozens of children displayed symptoms of the infection and needed immediate hospitalization, thus overtaxing the hospital's isolation facilities and pushing the nursing staff to the limits of their capacity. No month proved more challenging than December 1914, when the Contagious Disease Hospital admitted 195 measles cases, the highest single-month total on record.[29] During that outbreak, Margaret found herself "filling in wherever and whenever called upon."[30] Even though Island 3 had its own chief nurse by this time, hired just a year earlier, Margaret's help was needed.

Peering out a window in the General Hospital, Margaret noticed some commotion along the walkway connecting the three islands. Male attendants rushed back and forth between the Great Hall in the Main Immigration Building and the Contagious Disease Hospital, carefully navigating the narrow path; some wheeled the hand ambulance while others cradled sheet-wrapped children in their arms. Margaret threw on her coat and made her way toward Island 3, stepping aside to allow a hand ambulance to pass her on the footbridge. Looking through the glass panel at the top of the cart, Margaret caught a glimpse of a child's face, the telltale red measles rash splattered across his forehead. She picked up her pace.

By the time she reached the isolation wards at the far end of the island, Margaret realized the nurses had already filled up the smaller units completely and were triaging new patients as they arrived. After offering her services, Margaret was sent to supervise Measles Ward H, the small pavilion closest to the isolation wards that had been designated to receive confirmed cases—essentially all patients exhibiting the eruption of red spots.[31] On the ward, she found two nurses and a ward maid busily tending to patients, taking vital signs and performing assessments to determine which children needed immediate care.

Glancing at each patient, Margaret recognized the classic symptoms of the acute measles infection. Aside from the characteristic rash in varying stages of progression, most of the children had red, watery eyes, runny noses, and coughs. She knew that the nurses would watch for any signs of pneumonia, the most serious and sometimes fatal complication of measles, particularly in the youngest of their patients. Judging by their flushed cheeks and shivering, Margaret knew many of the children were already feverish; she made a note to find extra blankets. She also prepared basins of water for the ward nurses to use when they gave the children cooling sponge baths.

Knowing the importance of environmental conditions for patients with measles, Margaret carefully cracked open a few windows to ensure fresh air flowed through the ward without causing any drafts. She also hung the room thermometer in easy view so she and the nurses could keep the ambient temperature at precisely 68 degrees. Finally, she made sure to draw the shades on the windows to protect the children's sensitive eyes from too much light.[32]

Checking supplies was the next item on her agenda. Margaret took inventory of the amount of 2 percent boric acid on hand to make cleaning solutions for the children's eyes and then checked to see if enough Brown's mixture was available in the event a physician ordered it to treat coughs that were "very troublesome."[33]

She also spoke with one of the laundresses about preparing extra nightgowns and sheets. A few days from now the children's skin would begin to peel and the nurses would need to change the beds frequently.[34] Finally, she called the diet kitchen to see if they had ordered more milk. In addition to their usual between-meal snacks of milk and crackers, the children would need extra servings of eggnog.[35]

The nursing care for the children during their first week of measles infection continued in much the same way. The nurses managed symptoms for their patient's comfort, ensured the children had adequate nutrition, and monitored them for any signs of complications.

As the acute stage waned and the children began to feel better, the nurses faced wards filled with the children's playful mischief and activity. German immigrant John Henry Wilberding, who was hospitalized for measles at the age of six, remembered some of the mischief he and his brother caused: "Well, with measles you're supposed to pull the curtains . . . the lights, they hurt your eyes . . . there was a contest between the nurses and two little boys whether they were up or down."[36] The children also needed physical activity. Scottish immigrant Thomas Allen recalled that he passed his time "jumping from one bed to the other."[37] To address the children's need for increased activity, the nurses took them on daily walks down the long central corridor that connected all the buildings. Ward maid Josephine Friedman remembered the children's favorite view from the southwest-facing windows, noting, "you couldn't see very much of it, but they really enjoyed seeing the Statue of Liberty."[38]

The nurses always followed the tailored treatment protocols for each patient, and the children remained in the hospital until they had completely recovered. No standing orders existed since USPHS physicians attended to every case "according to its individual necessities."[39] While the state of New York mandated a minimum ten-day period of isolation for all measles cases, protocols in the Contagious Disease Hospital directed that patients stay on the wards until all their symptoms, including any complications like bronchitis, had resolved.[40] The USPHS physicians did not order the longer hospital stay out of fear that the patient remained infectious, but rather because they felt it was "in the interest of the patient" to ensure they had fully recuperated.[41]

Even in the rush of handling all those admissions, the nurses in the Contagious Disease Hospital not only maintained the strict procedures for isolation

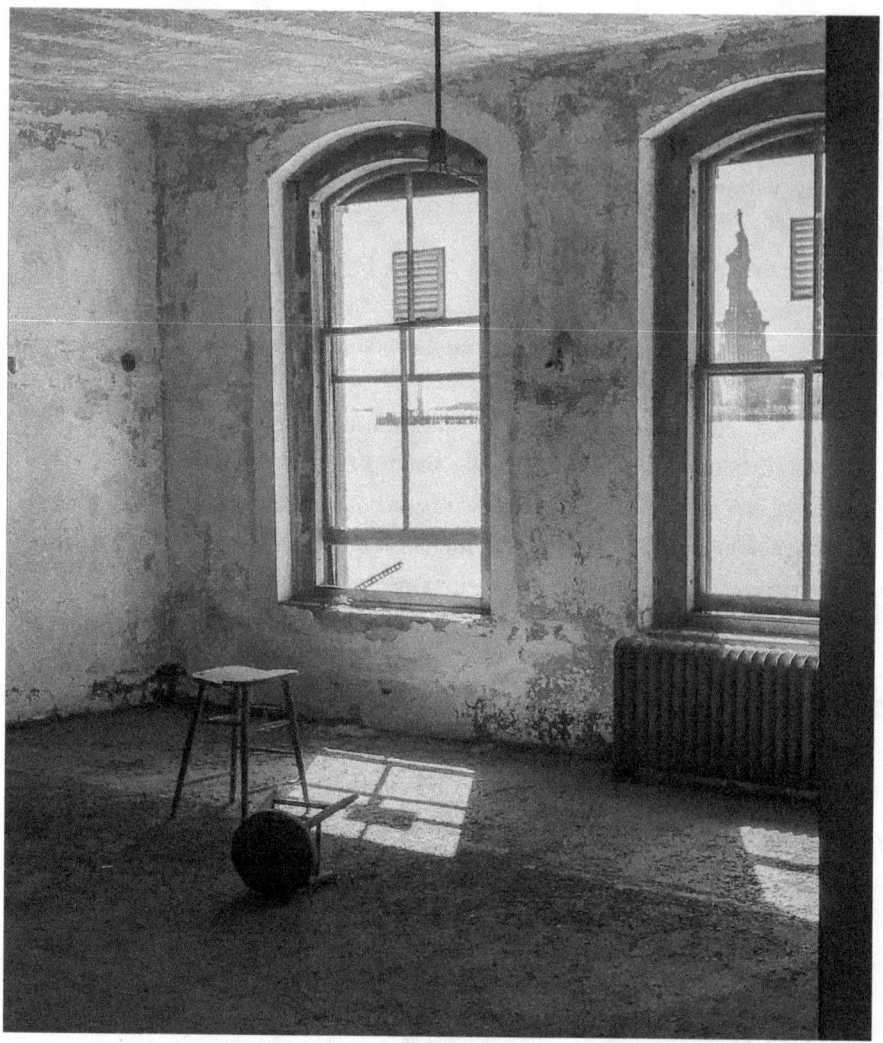

View of the Statue of Liberty through the window of a ward
in the Contagious Disease Hospital on Ellis Island.
Courtesy of Michelle C. Hehman, personal collection.

and infection prevention but also followed the well-established measles treat-ment protocols ordered by USPHS physicians. As a result of that diligent nursing care, the measles mortality rate for December 1914 was kept at only 5 percent.[42] The success, of course, was partly because of the camaraderie and teamwork employed "by the hospital staff under trying conditions."[43]

THE PROBLEM OF CLASS A CONDITIONS

The Contagious Disease Hospital didn't always run at full capacity. In fact, the variable and unpredictable nature of the daily admissions and total number of patients meant several wards or even entire buildings on Island 3 occasionally sat empty. Once they became aware of this fact, the USPHS physicians began to use the new hospital as overflow bedspace when the General Hospital was full. In fact, the unique design of the Contagious Disease Hospital made it an ideal facility to treat immigrants suffering from a variety of loathsome contagious diseases, including ringworm, hookworm, favus, and trachoma.[44]

Labeled as Class A conditions, these chronic illnesses warranted deportation under federal law; any immigrant certified with one of them would be prohibited from entering the United States. Immigrants could, however, ask to be treated for their Class A condition in one of the Ellis Island hospitals if they were willing and able to pay for their care. Very few petitions for medical treatment were denied, but many patients were eventually deported for unpaid hospital expenses.[45]

The patients diagnosed with Class A conditions presented a unique challenge for the nursing staff once Congress passed the Immigration Act of 1891. This act mandated that USPHS personnel inspect immigrants to determine eligibility to land and to care for any sick immigrants in the hospitals on Ellis Island. Thus, the nurses and physicians on Ellis Island were left to balance their responsibility to enforce immigration laws while simultaneously adhering to their ethical duty to individual patients. Although they did not take part in the Line inspection process, Margaret and other nurses frequently cared for immigrants—sometimes for weeks, months, and even years—who were ultimately deported because they suffered from mandatory excludable conditions under the prevailing federal law. This was particularly true for patients suffering from favus and trachoma.

CARING FOR CHILDREN WITH FAVUS

Favus, a severe and chronic inflammatory disease of the scalp, was one of the most common and easily diagnosable Class A conditions that physicians identified during the medical inspection process, owing largely to its distinctive and highly visible presentation. Caused by the fungus *Trichophyton schoenleinii*, "favus," from the Latin word for "honeycomb," was characterized by yellow, cup-shaped crusts that formed in dense masses around hair follicles. Patients usually complained of itching and burning of the scalp. Well-developed favus cases exhibited a characteristic odor "likened to musty straw or mice."[46] The disease primarily affected children, and if left untreated, progressed to involve larger areas of the scalp; as the crusts coalesced the affected hair would fall out, causing extensive permanent hair loss, skin atrophy, and scarring. Although chronic and nonfatal, the contagious nature and permanent sequelae of favus pushed US immigration officials to prevent its introduction and spread. As Immigration Commissioner Terence V. Powderly explained in 1902, "That death does not follow contact is no reason why we should invite it to our shores . . . if we remain indifferent simply because these diseases do not prove fatal to life, we evade our duty; for the health of the nation is imperilled [*sic*] when one man is diseased."[47]

The treatment for favus was lengthy and somewhat traumatic, especially for pediatric patients. When Line inspectors identified a new case, they directed an attendant to escort the immigrant directly to Ward D, the pavilion right next to the Contagious Disease Hospital's central administration building. Previously, that ward had been used for measles cases, but now it was needed to treat patients with favus and other loathsome contagious illnesses.[48]

Margaret came to dislike the painstaking primary treatment process for a new favus case because it added so much distress to an already intense day for

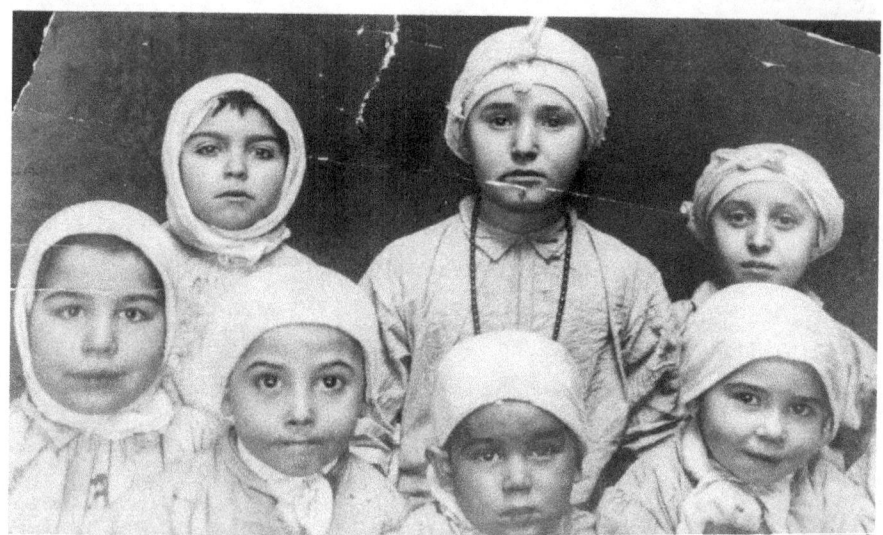

Immigrant children being treated for favus at the Ellis Island hospitals.
Courtesy of the National Park Service, Statue of Liberty National Monument.

the children. However, her time with the children offered her an opportunity to build rapport with patients who would be hospitalized for quite a while. Meeting her patients in the common bathroom, Margaret and her ward maid first cut their hair very short to be able to see the affected area more easily. Then they applied oil directly to the scalp and covered the child's head with a cap. While they waited for the oil to soften the favus crusts, Margaret and the ward maid inventoried the patient's belongings, tied them up in a burlap bag, and sent everything to the sterilization room. Then they gave their patient a thorough bath; when the bath was completed they removed the hood. By this time, the larger crusts were easy to lift off and "the remnants removed by thorough cleansing with soap and water."[49]

The next step in the treatment protocol proved to be the most difficult, particularly for patients who could not understand what was happening, either due to their young age or a language barrier. For the best outcomes, the nurses needed to extract all the patient's affected hair, not simply shave it off, so that the topical treatments could enter the open hair follicles. Margaret preferred an epilation method whereby she grasped the hair between her thumb and forefinger, covered with "a worn (roughened) kid glove finger cut from an old glove."[50] She then pulled gently until the affected and loosened hairs fell out. Next, she applied a mixture of carbolic acid and balsam of Peru, an antiseptic with the pleasant aroma of vanilla to counter the putrid smells coming from the now open pustules. Finally, Margaret applied boric acid powder and cod liver oil to the child's scalp and then covered their head in a white cotton handkerchief and gauze. Patients wore these protective bandages over their scalp "during the entire hospitalization."[51] Nurses checked the scalp daily and extracted new crusts and any additional diseased hairs "as long as found in any number, and occasionally thereafter" until a cure was "effected."[52] The treatment for favus could take months, and though remission was likely, a full cure was not always achieved. Immigrants hospitalized with favus, however, had a much greater chance of eventually being admitted into the United States than individuals suffering from trachoma.

THE CHALLENGE OF TRACHOMA

Trachoma, a highly contagious disease of the eye, was a particularly challenging health problem in the early twentieth century. The disease, whose name comes from the Greek word for "rough," caused chronic inflammation of the inner eye-lid, leading to areas of granulation, scarring, and ulceration of the eyeball. Left untreated, trachoma ultimately led to blindness. Easily transmissible through a person's touch and direct personal contact, trachoma was considered a "menace" because of its highly contagious nature and the "seriousness of its sequelae."[53] In 1897 trachoma became the first disease officially classified as "dangerous contagious" by Surgeon General Walter S. Wyman, thereby "making mandatory the deportation of all arriving aliens who are afflictted."[54] But now that the Contagious Disease Hospital had additional bed space and appropriate isolation facilities, the USPHS could offer treatment to more patients with trachoma.

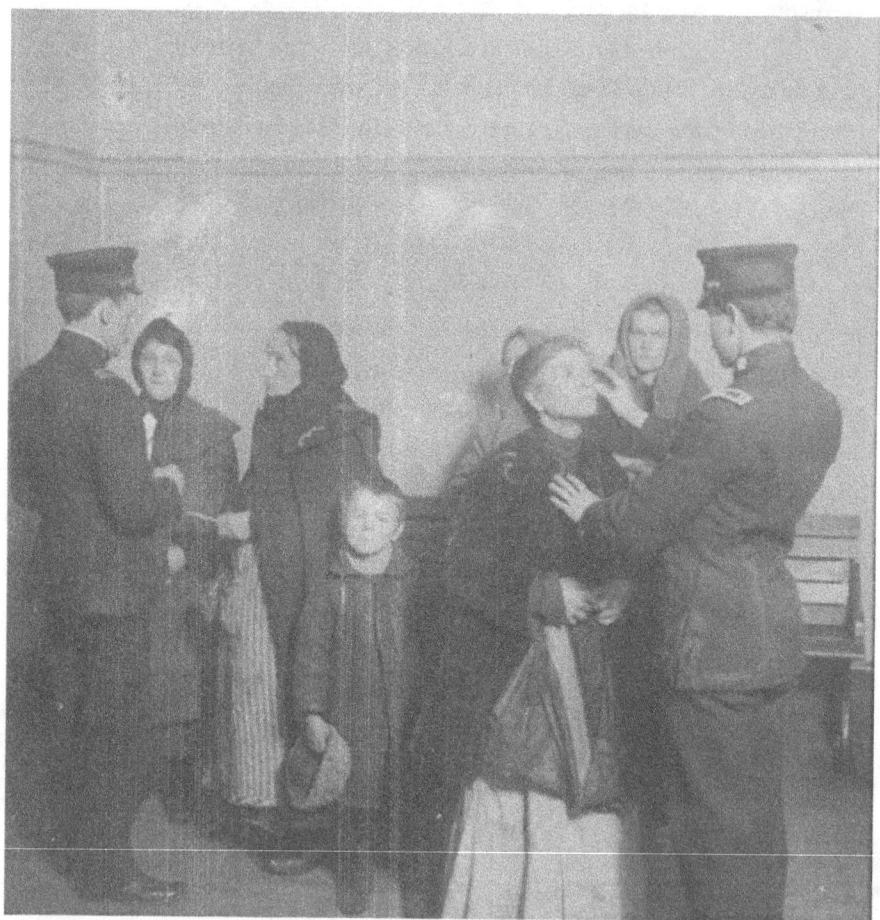

Trachoma inspection of female immigrants at Ellis Island, circa 1911.
Courtesy of the Library of Congress, Prints and Photographs Online Catalog.

Whenever Margaret encountered a newly admitted patient with a chalk *Ct* (contagious trachoma) on their lapel, she steeled herself for the challenge ahead and counseled other nurses to do the same. Trachoma cases were almost as difficult to handle emotionally as they were clinically. For these patients, a long and grueling course of treatment lay ahead with very little possibility of success. On Ellis Island, the average hospital stay for trachoma was about six months, with approximately 95 percent of these patients eventually deported to their home country.[55] Margaret knew that few cases of well-defined trachoma were "ever cured," but she and the other nurses maintained hope as they diligently carried out the prescribed treatment regimen.[56]

The hospital admission of patients with trachoma followed a predictable course. The patient initially remained in an isolation ward for a one- to two-week observation stage while their diagnosis was confirmed. Then they received maintenance treatments on a weekly basis. As soon as Margaret finished general admission procedures for her trachoma patients, she settled them into a dark room and began a strict schedule of cold applications, irrigations, and eye washes. Her only goal during the initial phase was "to reduce the inflammatory symptoms as soon as possible" so that a physician could make a proper diagnosis.[57] She applied cold compresses over her patient's eyes for two hours at a time, with an hour break in between. Three times a day, following the compress treatment, Margaret instilled an antiseptic 20 percent argyrol solution directly into her patient's eye. To reduce the risk of transmission, she carefully washed away any eye secretions using a 4 percent boric acid solution, all the while remembering to thoroughly scrub and disinfect her own hands and any other surfaces around the patient.[58]

Once the physician made a definitive diagnosis of trachoma, Margaret assisted patients with the maintenance phase of treatment. While Margaret ensured that her patients had "hygienic surroundings, plenty of fresh air, and a nutritious diet," the USPHS physicians employed various invasive procedures to "prevent or restrict as far as possible" the corneal damage that led to blindness.[59] Once a week, Margaret escorted her trachoma patients to the operating room on Island 3, where they endured follicular expression, grattage, and/or blue stone treatment.[60] The procedures were painful and traumatic, involving the manual rupture and expression of trachoma follicles on the conjunctiva, scrubbing the eyelids with a toothbrush dipped in antiseptic, and directly applying a corrosive copper sulfate crystal (blue stone) to the diseased areas. Although patients received a topical cocaine anesthetic, they remained awake during the treatment. Fifteen-year-old Josephine Calloway received eleven months of trachoma treatments on Ellis Island and remembered that "they used to use silver nitrate and blue stone. They used to rub the lids, turn the lids inside out and burn . . . I had scars from the tears for at least five years."[61] Josephine was "one of the lucky ones," discharged home to her parents in Brooklyn after the USPHS physicians declared her cured.[62] Most trachoma patients were not so fortunate.

Margaret watched as most of the immigrants with trachoma were barred from entering the United States after months of painful treatments. She recalled the tragedy of that reality, noting:

> It was especially hard to witness the separation of families when perhaps
> the hopes of a lifetime were shattered. Among other cases this happened
> when a man who had come to the United States, saved a little money,
> established a home for his wife and children and brought them over,
> only to find, however, that one of them was suffering from trachoma.
> Deportation was mandatory and the husband was helpless. Sometimes
> he would keep the children who were eligible to land and the certified
> sufferer, whether wife or child, had to return. Deportations of this sort
> furnished the most moving and tragic scenes one can imagine.[63]

BALANCING POLICY AND PLACE

Navigating professional responsibilities on Ellis Island meant that the nurses had to confront the duality of their roles—agents of the state on the one hand and professional healers on the other. According to personal accounts from the USPHS physicians and nurses, the two professions handled the potential conflict in entirely different ways: the physicians separated the tasks and responsibilities of their competing roles by assigning some doctors to Line inspection and others to the hospital, while the nurses integrated their various responsibilities and accepted the fact that their serving both patient and country would involve joy and pain.

The administrative structure of Ellis Island provided the USPHS physicians with organizational separation between their many roles. The Boarding and Inspection Division performed medical examinations on the Line, and the Medical Division worked in the hospital caring for admitted patients. Physicians were assigned to either division for a specified time period, switched back and forth as was needed or required, but were never involved in both simultaneously. This allowed the physicians to focus on a single set of responsibilities associated with their current assignment and compartmentalize the multiple roles they fulfilled.

The Line inspection process almost certainly caused the greatest turmoil for the physicians, who knew that a medical certificate was often the sole evidence used by the Board of Special Inquiry to deny entrance to new immigrants. Dr. Gertrude Slaughter, one of the few female USPHS physicians inspecting immigrants at Ellis Island later recalled that turmoil: "I approached my task with considerable misgiving, feeling that I had become part of the crushing mechanism."[64] However, the separation of the Public Health Service from the Board of Special Inquiry may have diffused much of the individual responsibility physicians felt in the deportation process. Physicians presented their objective findings in the form of a medical certificate, and the Board of Special Inquiry used that information as they saw fit. Since USPHS physicians were specifically precluded from serving on the Board of Special Inquiry, they were never directly involved in the final decision or appeals process for deportation cases. As Dr. Grover Kempf remembered, "I never heard any of the medical officers discuss immigration laws. That was something that was not in our line and there was no indication of the need of discussing [them]. We did what we thought was right."[65]

Nurses, on the other hand, did not have the ability to separate themselves from the controversy that sometimes arose when serving the best interests of the country meant crushing the dreams of a patient. To balance the sorrow, Margaret and her fellow nurses focused on the moments of joy that also came with working in the Ellis Island hospitals—the many births they attended, the remarkable recoveries they witnessed, and their patients' responses to the nurses' kindness. Guided by Immigration Commissioner William Williams, who insisted in 1902 that "immigrants were to be treated with kindness and civility by everyone on Ellis Island," nurses made the biggest impact on the immigrants, as they had prolonged and direct contact with those who were the most vulnerable.[66] The nurses' attempts paid off. One immigrant later recalled, "The nurses, the ladies in white . . . were very nice. They talked to the children. They stroked their hair, and they touched their cheeks."[67] Another later recalled, "Miss Hannah, oh, she was so good. . . . She'd always bring me a present from New York City when she'd come back. . . . I had a doll and some leather gloves."[68]

Notions of discipline, self-sacrifice, and duty, often cultivated and ingrained in nurses since the early days of their training, provided the foundation for much of their practice, with some nurses even willing to risk their own safety to help immigrant patients. In late October 1913, Nurse Anna Olsen saved the life of her patient Marthe Novik, who, in a state of delirium from scarlet fever, escaped from the ward and jumped off the dock into the harbor. Displaying "pluck and devotion," Anna "without hesitancy jumped into the water after her and succeeded in swimming with her to one of the piles on the face of the dock."[69] Though a substantial increase in pay was requested for her "heroic conduct," no raise was granted since Anna had not taken on additional duties or displayed new capabilities.[70] Ellis Island nurses were expected to be completely devoted to their patients.

Thus, the work of nursing on Ellis Island involved navigating a professional middle space, in which the nurses' roles demanded a great deal of responsibility with little commensurate control over outcomes. Margaret and the rest of the nurses found themselves bearing witness to the full range of the human experience, knowing that the island was "a place of hopes and tears, of jubilations and disappointments."[71] In trying times, Margaret turned to her Catholic faith for comfort, giving "gratitude to the Almighty" for the "precious opportunity" to serve as a nurse at the Ellis Island General Hospital.[72]

CHANGES IN WARTIME

Just as nursing policies and immigration procedures on Ellis Island became more standardized, global geopolitical events in the mid-1910s brought major changes. Margaret immediately felt the different atmosphere on the island, commenting, "Late in the summer of 1914 the Great War burst like a volcano on the world. It had an instant effect on immigration."[73] As the conflict in Europe intensified, overall rates of immigration through Ellis Island dramatically slowed. In 1915, the commissioner general commented that "the past year has been unique in the history of immigration . . . the world was shocked and amazed at the opening of a conflict which soon involved, directly or indirectly, practically every country from which our heaviest immigration has come in recent decades."[74] More than eight hundred thousand immigrants had passed through Ellis Island in 1914; the following three years saw annual rates below two hundred thousand.[75]

With fewer arrivals to process each day, the USPHS officers had time to perform more thorough medical inspections, but they found deporting any new arrivals was more difficult as fewer steamship companies were willing to risk a journey across the Atlantic during the war. That decrease in deportations was an unexpected boon for immigrant patients diagnosed with a traditionally excludable condition like favus or trachoma. Now patients had more time to allow the protracted treatments for these diseases to be successful. As a result, in the first few years of the Great War, many immigrants with favus and trachoma were eventually declared "cured" and allowed to enter the United States.

The Ellis Island nurses initially welcomed the decreased number of new admissions and the opportunity to keep patients in the hospital while they recovered completely. In fact, as Margaret noted, "For a short time the hospital staff at Ellis Island had a breathing spell affording a little relaxation which was sorely needed."[76] However, the nurses' respite "did not last long."[77] Within weeks of the United States entering the Great War, the government made major changes to how the island was used.

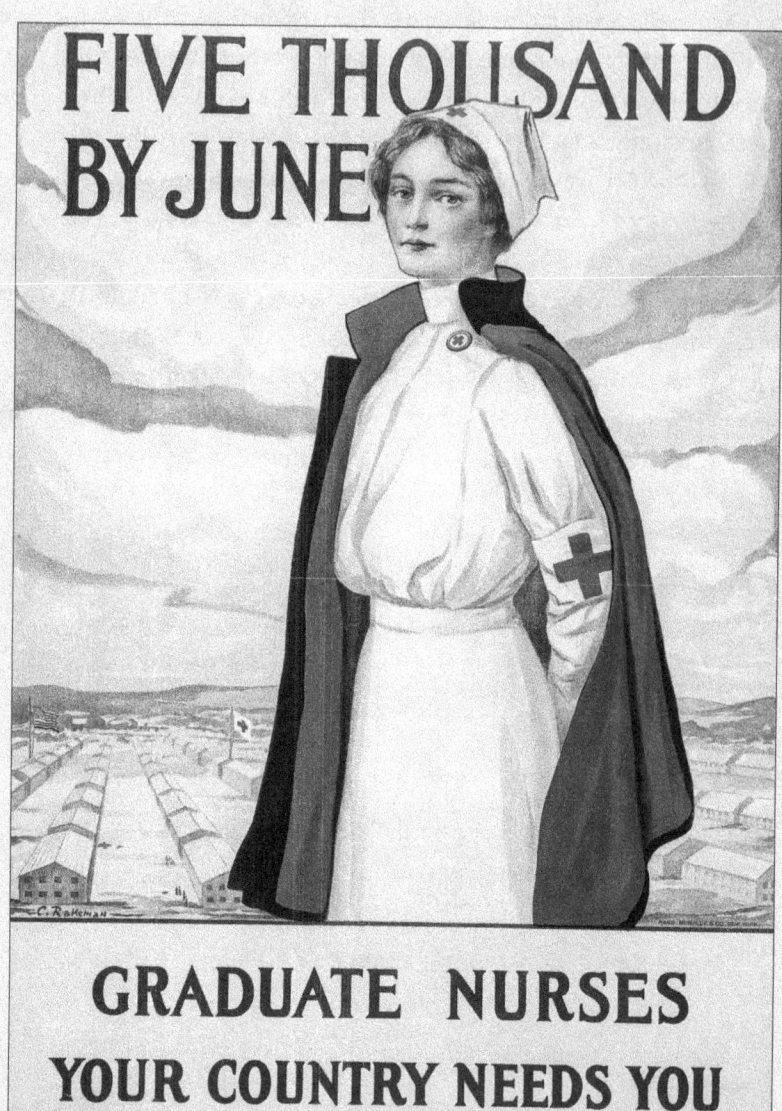

"Five Thousand by June" graduate nurse recruitment poster, 1917.
Courtesy of the Library of Congress, Prints and Photographs Online Catalog.

CHAPTER 4

NURSES ON ELLIS ISLAND DURING WORLD WAR I 1917–1919

Those were stirring times at the Island . . .
The air was tense with unrest.

MARGARET V. DALY[1]

W ithin a few weeks of the United States declaring war on Germany in April 1917, Margaret Daly's role as chief nurse of the Ellis Island General Hospital changed dramatically. Making rounds of the wards in mid-June, Margaret stopped and surveyed the scene. No longer were the beds filled with immigrants; the few who had managed to escape the war and sail across the Atlantic to the United States were now inspected in other locations around New York Harbor. Others entered at different US ports, like Angel Island in San Francisco, California, and Pelican Island in Galveston, Texas.[2] Meanwhile, on Ellis Island the hospital beds were now occupied by German prisoners of war who had fallen ill, captured enemy sea merchants who were sick or injured, and US coastguardsmen and their family members who needed care. As members of the groups being housed on the island during the war, all were entitled to receive treatment at the hospital.

Given that diverse mix of patients, the atmosphere in the Ellis Island General Hospital was strained. Sighing deeply, Margaret realized how challenging it would be to care for "enemy aliens" right alongside US coastguardsmen and other military men: "One felt that turmoil and violence might result at any moment. . . . Think of it! Enemy aliens, coastguardsmen, and militia, all commingled in the same hospital."[3] She and her staff would have to balance their professional "duty to care"—regardless of a patient's nationality and politics—with their patriotic duty to their country.[4] She would have to speak to her nurses about that.

Surveying the room, Margaret added another agenda item for that talk with the nurses. She would have to remind them to be careful not to say anything of military importance that could get back to the enemy. Even the slightest bit of information could have dire consequences for national security. As she later recalled, "We had to be constantly on the alert and guard our speech, as there might be spies amongst us."[5]

Exercising caution in their conversations would not be the nurses' only concern. Although Margaret was not yet aware of all the dangers that could occur, it would later become clear that the nurses also had to protect patients from immediate threats to their safety. Ward 1, designated for women and children, was of special concern, given the fact that so many military men were on the island. Later Margaret documented one particularly troubling incident, writing, "One time a drunken soldier entered the ward and pointed a loaded rifle at each of the patients in succession, frightening them out of their wits. We had quite a task to calm the women and children and to get the drunken intruder out of their sight."[6]

In June 1917, however, that incident had not yet happened, and Margaret was happily unaware that it would. Glancing out a back window toward Island 3, Margaret considered the other changes that would occur on Ellis Island now that the country was at war. Chief among these was the fact that the US Army had just appropriated the Contagious Disease Hospital for the mobilization of hundreds of newly recruited army nurses. Margaret had already been informed that Edith Agnes Mury, former assistant superintendent of nursing in the United States Army Nurse Corps, would arrive on June 17 to take over the command of those nurses before they departed for Europe. Hopefully she and Miss Mury would get along. Even though they would have completely different assignments on two different parts of Ellis Island, the pair certainly couldn't avoid interacting on occasion. Perhaps she should invite Miss Mury to tea so they could become acquainted. She should at least make the attempt. She had much to tell the army nurse leader about living and working on Ellis Island. At this point Margaret was not at all sure she wanted another chief nurse on the island, or for that matter, a score of young army nurses stationed there—even if they would be strictly confined to Island 3.

Actually, Margaret had to admit that the US Army's plan to mobilize nurses from Ellis Island made sense. The army's need for a mobilization site, the island's location, and the fact that its hospitals had been underutilized since the start of the war in Europe in 1914 made Ellis Island the ideal spot for military use.

Clearly the army needed a mobilization site for nurses. For over a year the US government had been preparing for the possibility of war and now it was a reality. Under the direction of the army's surgeon general, teams of physicians and nurses from across the country had been organizing a reserve corps of fifty Base Hospitals to which the country could turn in the event the United States was drawn into the European conflict.[7] Each Base Hospital had a staff of 27 medical officers, at least 60 nurses, and 153 enlisted men.[8] By April 1917 when the United States declared war on Germany, thirty-three Base Hospital units were almost ready to deploy overseas. To complete that process, members of those units required uniforms, equipment, passports, vaccines, and basic military training.[9] The government now had to find locations on the East Coast where those final preparations could be made. Within a matter of weeks, US Army officials decided to house American Red Cross nurses on Ellis Island; physicians and enlisted men would be mustered in military camps surrounding the Upper Bay.[10]

The geographic location of the island played a significant role in the government's decision. With its proximity to other military camps, nearby factories and supply depots, and the Atlantic Ocean, Ellis Island was perfectly situated for its new mission. Soldiers from the surrounding camps could teach the nurses the basics of military life, including how to salute and march in formation; factories, supply depots, and stores in Manhattan could easily equip nurses with uniforms and boots; and ferries could transport the nurses to nearby wharfs where they would board troop ships for the voyage overseas.

The fact that the buildings on the island had been underutilized for years also played a part in the army's decision. Since the beginning of the Great War in Europe in 1914, the numbers of European immigrants arriving at the Port of New York had sharply decreased, resulting in fewer steerage-class passengers coming through Ellis Island.[11] As a result, many of the hospital beds in various Ellis Island hospitals remained unoccupied. In 1917 it was reasonable to use the Great Hall in the Main Immigration Building for US Army offices and the empty wards of the Contagious Disease Hospital on Island 3 as dormitories for Red Cross Army nurses awaiting transport to Europe.

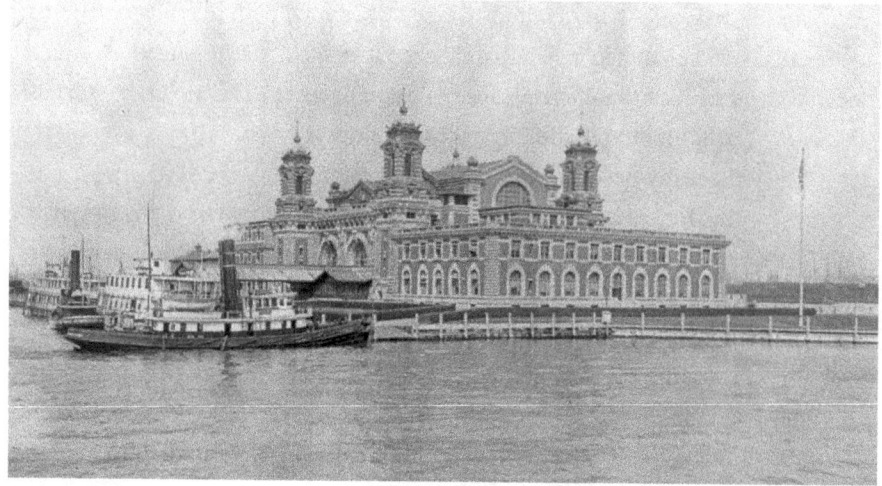

View of Ellis Island from New York harbor, 1917.
Courtesy of the Library of Congress, Prints and Photographs Online Catalog.

EDITH AGNES MURY

Sailing across the Upper Bay on June 17, 1917, with her newly appointed assistant Mina Keenan, Edith Agnes Mury contemplated her new assignment as chief nurse of the Army Nurse Corps mobilization station on Ellis Island. It would be a very busy summer. For the moment, however, she was determined to enjoy this brief interlude on the ferry. Luckily her cap was pinned firmly in place; the wind had picked up as the ferry made its way across the bay. Edith took a deep breath and smiled. She loved the feeling of the cool air against her face, the view of the Statue of Liberty, and the sight of the Manhattan skyline fading in the distance. Besides, she enjoyed the bustling activity of the harbor. She had not been surrounded by this much water—or for that matter, this many battleships— since her tour of duty in the Navy Nurse Corps before being transferred to the US Army a year earlier.[12] She should just relax and enjoy the moment. Sitting back on the bench, she did so for a few minutes, then leaned forward to take her pen and tiny notepad from her purse—her propensity for efficiency forcing her to use every available moment. Her mind was racing with all she had to do. First, she had to set up her office; then she had to repurpose the Contagious Disease Hospital wards to accommodate nurses rather than patients.[13] Hopefully, she'd have a few weeks to do so. For now, however, she'd at least jot down a list of priorities.

Then she would check the dining facilities and order food from the quartermaster. She would also have to discuss the division of responsibilities with Mina Keenan, and finally, introduce herself to Margaret Daly. No doubt Miss Daly would have some advice for her about the logistics of living and working on an island.

Continuing to put her thoughts on paper, Edith noted that she had to arrange for the nurses to be photographed for their passports, receive their vaccinations, and obtain their uniforms, boots, and other equipment. She was glad she could rely on Mina to assign the nurses to their quarters and ensure they had everything they needed. She herself would handle the office work.[14]

Within a few minutes, the ferry's landing at the dock jolted Edith from her thoughts. Getting up from her seat, she made her way to the bow and down the gangplank. Turning right, she headed to Island 1. She dropped off some papers in her new office in the Main Immigration Building, met the stenographer who was assigned to help her, and saw if she could find any information about the arrival dates for the nurses.[15] She needed a cup of tea!

Edith's plans for taking a few days to get organized were short-lived. No sooner had she entered the Great Hall than she received a telegram stating that "66 nurses would arrive the next day."[16] That was not the only disturbing news, however. She was also notified that the wards in the Contagious Disease Hospital were not only dirty but completely empty. She had less than twenty-four hours to convert some of them into dormitories for the Red Cross Army nurses.[17] Her tea would have to wait.

Setting to work immediately, Edith called the quartermaster and ordered "beds, bedding, and a few accessories" to be brought by tugs from the Supply Depot in New York City. She then arranged for infantrymen from Governors Island to clean the wards and set up the sleeping quarters. Each nurse was assigned a single bed, a chair, and a small bedside table. A "T" bar at the head of each bed served for hanging their uniforms, dresses, and coats. As Edith later recalled, "When the nurses arrived the next day, they had clean white hospital beds but little else."[18] Indeed, the stark living quarters, one communal bathroom for each ward, and a multitude of army regulations would soon have the nurses adjusting to the realities of life in the military.[19]

Over the next two weeks, assisted by Mina, Edith established a system to process the nurses' papers and facilitate their assimilation into the Army Nurse

Corps. That system was efficient.[20] As Edith later recalled, "Men of the Hospital Corps met the nurses at the train depot and escorted them" to Battery Park to board the ferry, while men with army trucks "obtained the nurses' baggage and sent it to us by boat."[21] Describing the process, she said:

> When the nurses arrived, they came single file through my office, where a sergeant, the stenographer, and I received their papers and secured such information as was necessary for our records. Miss Keenan then took them in charge and gave them beds and mess assignments at the immigration dining room.[22]

Following that, the new recruits made their way across the narrow wooden bridge to the Contagious Disease Hospital dormitories on Island 3, no doubt relieved to have survived their first few hours.

SARAH PARSONS AND BASE HOSPITAL 6

On June 30, 1917, just thirteen days after Edith took charge and welcomed the first group of army nurses to her command, sixty-four nurses from Base Hospital 6 boarded the ferry for Ellis Island. The group, sponsored by Boston's Massachusetts General Hospital, was led by Sarah Parsons, superintendent of nursing at Massachusetts General Hospital Training School for Nurses.[23] A woman of "practical and energetic temperament, with snapping gray eyes," Sarah would rely on her longstanding relationships with the nurses she had formerly supervised at Massachusetts General Hospital to enhance an esprit de corps among her new recruits.[24]

Responding to the tense expressions on the nurses' faces, Sarah smiled, trying to assure them that

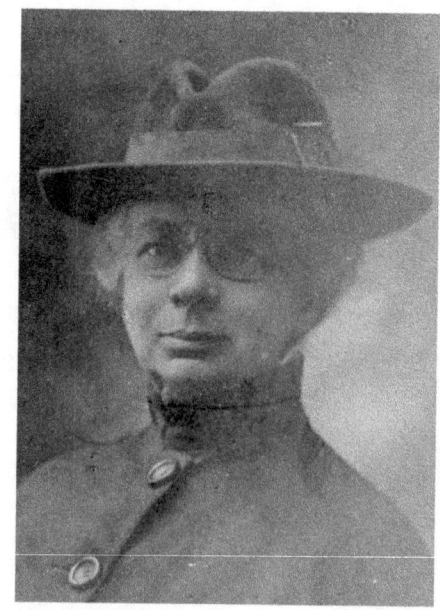

Sarah Parsons.
Courtesy of the Massachusetts General Hospital Archives.

all would be well. She knew that the young women were excited about what lay ahead, but also that they were anxious about what it would be like to be in the army. No doubt the young women were also tired from the preparations of the past month. Their unit had received orders to activate in late May, then had waited for several weeks before receiving further directives to proceed to Ellis Island.[25] Those weeks had been a whirlwind of activity. First they had the swearing in, then they rolled twenty-five hundred bandages that "had to be ready immediately," later they packed their steamer trunks, and finally said a series of goodbyes to friends and families.[26] Of course the new recruits were tired and full of mixed emotions.[27]

Before Sarah worried any further about how her nurses were coping, the ferry docked on Ellis Island and the nurses disembarked en masse, not yet having been taught how to march in an orderly fashion. That lesson would come soon. During their time on the island, a US Army sergeant would drill the nurses "in the rudiments of military formations."[28]

For now, the nurses proceeded to the chief nurse's office in the Great Hall and began to experience what it meant to be a member of the Red Cross Army Nurse Corps.[29] First, they completed a plethora of military forms and received their bed assignments. Over the next few days, they received passports and uniforms along with lectures on the army regulations they were required to follow.[30]

Their time on the island was short, hardly enough for the Base Hospital 6 nurses to be photographed for their passports and fitted for outerwear and boots. On July 11, 1917, less than two weeks after their arrival, the nurses joined the men of their unit for the transatlantic crossing.[31] Aboard the RMS *Aurania*, they completed their orientation by participating in emergency drills, attending French classes, and learning military etiquette.[32]

BECOMING AN ARMY NURSE

Part of the nurses' incorporation into the Red Cross Army Nurse Corps involved the adoption of the army nurse uniform. From April until late August 1917, each nurse was given only the outdoor uniform—a blue serge Norfolk coat and skirt along with brown leather boots. Until the army adopted an official "indoor" outfit, the nurses were allowed to wear their own traditional white uniforms and caps. That policy was short-lived, however. On August 27, 1917, the War Department issued orders specifying that nurses "conform in all respects" and adopt both indoor and outdoor regulation army uniforms. For "general ward duty overseas," the uniform was a gray cotton dress covered with a white apron.[33] Despite their distaste for the drab, utilitarian uniforms, the nurses complied. They had no choice in the matter.

By the end of August, more than seven hundred nurses had adopted the army regulation uniforms, completed their paperwork, and were considered full-fledged army nurses. Several units had already left for France. By September, new recruits were arriving on Ellis Island.[34]

ELSIE BLANCHE AUGUSTINE AND COLLEAGUES, BASE HOSPITAL 23

Elsie Blanche Augustine, an army reserve nurse from upstate New York, was one of many nurses boarding the ferry for Ellis Island in September 1917. The thirty-two-year-old had enlisted in the US Army Nurse Corps earlier in the summer with five other nurses from Buffalo. In August, the group had received their active-duty orders directing them to Ellis Island "for mobilization and to await convoy to France" with Base Hospital 23.[35]

After checking her purse one more time to make sure she had the orders with her, Blanche (as she preferred to be called) looked up and grinned at her friends, Evelyn Carney and Martha Morningstar. They were really on their way. Think of it! First, they would be stationed on Ellis Island just a short distance from Manhattan, where they could shop and sightsee. Blanche especially wanted to visit the Statue of Liberty sometime soon. Then they would cross the Atlantic on a huge ocean liner filled with thousands of soldiers. She had never experienced anything like this in Buffalo!

Exiting the ferry just minutes later, the three nurses made their way through registration and then on to their quarters on Island 3. After unpacking they hoped they might have time to sit on the quay and enjoy the view before it was time for dinner and bed. The next morning, their new life would begin.

For Blanche and her friends, their days on Ellis Island soon settled into a predictable routine; part military and part civilian life. Breakfast included coffee and "the usual eggs and fried potatoes" in the staff dining room—the menu typical of home, the setting quite different. The "mandatory roll call" occurred at 9:00 a.m., as each nurse had to be accounted for once a day.[36] For the first few weeks, after roll call Blanche and her colleagues often took the ferry into Manhattan to shop, attend services at Trinity Episcopal Church, or have lunch or dinner at various restaurants, their favorites being Riggs, the Waldorf-Astoria, and Childs. Becoming accustomed to the "hurry up and wait" aspects of military life, the new recruits passed long afternoons watching movies at Lowe's Victoria Theatre and attending Broadway shows. Enjoying their last days of freedom, Blanche and her friends visited the aquarium at Battery Park, took boat trips around Manhattan, and sailed up the Hudson River to Bear Mountain. Because they never knew when their sailing orders might arrive, the nurses were not allowed to stay in the city overnight. Trying to comply with these orders, they often rushed downtown to catch the late-night ferry back to the island.[37]

On the island, the nurses could not escape the fact that the country was at war. As Chief Nurse Edith Mury observed, "All the activities of a harbor given over to war went on in our front yard." Moreover, she noted, "a thousand interned Germans and imprisoned German agents under heavy guard" were on the island, their presence producing "a shadow of apprehension."[38]

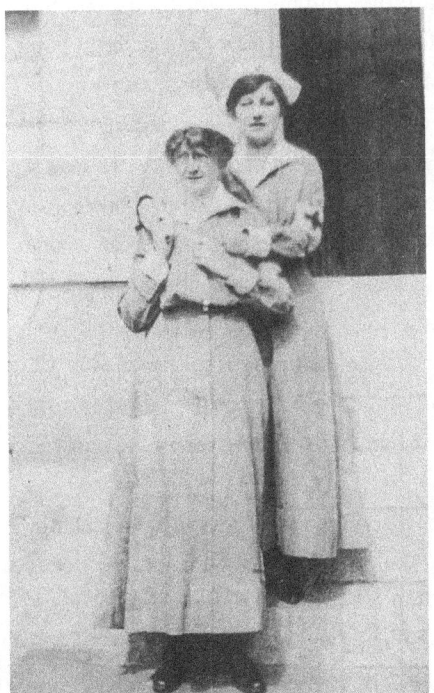

E. Blanche Augustine and Evelyn Carney,
circa 1917.
Courtesy of the Digital Collections,
University at Buffalo Libraries.

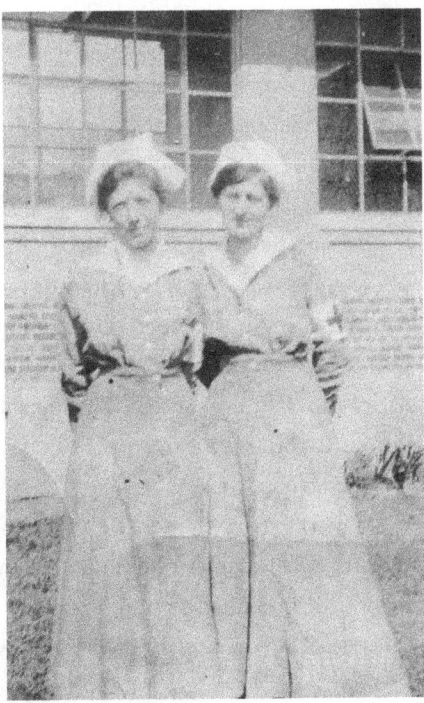

E. Blanche Augustine with
Martha Morningstar, circa 1917.
Courtesy of the Digital Collections,
University at Buffalo Libraries.

Thus, on Ellis Island the reality of the nurses' new life in the military took hold. As the days progressed towards their date of departure, Buffalo's Base Hospital 23 nurses had fewer and fewer hours of free time. They had much to do to be ready to serve in a foreign country. Like those who had preceded them, Blanche and her colleagues completed paperwork, attended French classes, memorized army regulations, and spent hours in military drills. Between classes, on sunny days the nurses often walked along the quay, observing the activities of the harbor. On "disagreeable rainy days," however, they stayed in their barracks, reading, writing letters, and waiting for their deployment orders.[39]

DELAYS AND DEPARTURES

Delays in embarkation were typical, primarily because there was an "acute shortage of American and Allied tonnage" and the transport of American combat troops and supplies took precedence over the nurses' departures.[40] Sometimes however, the delays were caused by problems obtaining equipment. Writing to National Headquarters in Washington, DC, on October 16, 1917, Director of the Red Cross Bureau of Nursing Clara Noyes asked for additional funds to ensure an adequate supply of equipment in the New York storeroom. Her request was a valid one. As hundreds of nurses prepared to embark for France, the director was finding it "increasingly difficult to secure sleeping bags, steamer trunks, rubber boots and slickers" on short notice. Providing Red Cross Headquarters with a specific example, she wrote, "We now have four units waiting in New York for sleeping bags."[41]

Clara Noyes was successful in her appeal. On October 30, 1917, the War Council appropriated $100,000 for the purchase of equipment specifically for US Army and Navy nurses. That appropriation would facilitate the process of getting nurses to the front. Now, the military just had to find room for nurses on the crowded troop ships.

When transport orders finally arrived, a serious mood pervaded the island. Writing in her diary on November 14, 1917, Maude Essig of Base Hospital 32 documented that reality: "Tuesday, in all day. A Unit is leaving, and all passes have been called in. [Our] greatest diversion today was French Class and scrubbing the floor."[42]

More often than not, final preparations were hurried, as army officials, concerned that giving out any information about the dates of sailing or the names of the ships would "jeopardize the lives of those on board," kept this information secret until the last possible moment.[43] Such was the case for the nurses of Base

Hospital 23. After two and a half months on Ellis Island, the nurses had less than twenty-four hours' notice to prepare for their departure, slated for November 22, 1917, to join their unit's officers and enlisted men in Jersey City before sailing.[44] Writing in her diary, Blanche Augustine documented the event: "Our last breakfast on Ellis Island. Such a horrid rainy day to start out but we're thankful we're going!"[45] In Jersey City, Blanche was fingerprinted for her certificate of identity. It was completed just in time; a few hours later she and her colleagues boarded the *Carpathian* for travel to France.

In early December 1917, the nurses of Indiana's Base Hospital 32 also left Ellis Island without much warning. According to Maude Essig, "December 3, 1917—Houser and I got in at 12:30 AM—found everyone packed or packing to leave for places unknown—for sure this time." The next morning, she and her unit embarked at 9:00 a.m., "everybody helping everyone else." The Ellis Island Restaurant people served them "coffee and sandwiches" after they boarded the quartermaster tug that took them to their transport ship, the USS *George Washington*.[46]

Less than two weeks later, the nurses of Base Hospital 34, organized by the Episcopal Hospital of Philadelphia, deployed. With their chief nurse Katherine Brown, the nurses joined the men of their unit on December 15 to sail across the Atlantic on the SS *Leviathan*, an ocean liner with the capacity to transport thousands of military personnel.[47] Having witnessed numerous departures from the island, Edith Mury described the typical scene:

> Shore leave was stopped, no communication with friends or relatives
> was allowed; trunks were inspected and locked and the unit stood by for
> the tug that was to take them to the transport. On arrival of the tug, the
> command "Fall in!" was given, followed by "Forward March!" and sixty-
> five silent, blue-clad white-faced women with chins well up and eyes to the
> front marched down the dock and onto the tug in soldierly formation.[48]

MORE DEPLOYMENTS IN THE WINTER OF 1918

As the war continued and the battles in Europe grew more intense, the demand for nurses increased. By January 1918 the US Army was calling for thousands of additional nurses to volunteer. Registered nurses from all over the United States responded. Included among these were University of Pennsylvania Base Hospital 20 nurses, who "one by one received orders to report to Ellis Island between January 15 and February 18, 1918."[49] Nurses from Base Hospital 3, organized by

Mt. Sinai Hospital in New York City, were also mobilized. Under the command of Chief Nurse Amy Trench, they arrived on Ellis Island on January 15, leaving on the *Lapland* only a few weeks later on February 8, 1918.

That winter hundreds of army nurses spent time on Ellis Island. Writing to the *American Journal of Nursing*, Jean Haviland later recounted her own and her friend's reaction to the experience: "We began to realize how small a 'bit' ours was after all, when we knew that we were only two out of hundreds constantly coming and going."[50]

The nurses' perception of the small part they played in the larger war effort was not unfounded. Indeed, there was a steady stream of energetic and excited young army nurses going on and off the island during the opening months of 1918. To accommodate the increase, dormitory space in the Contagious Disease Hospital had been expanded. By the winter of 1918, bed capacity in the nurses' dorms had doubled from 250 to 500 beds.[51]

Being crowded into dormitories, sharing communal bathrooms, and eating in a cafeteria provided the nurses only a glimpse of the reality of army life,

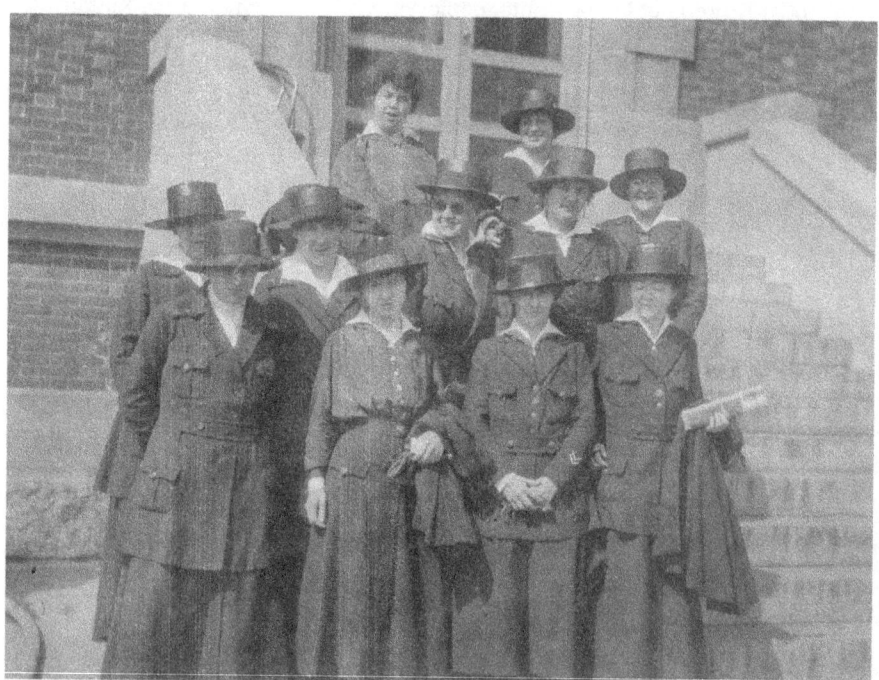

Army nurses in uniform on Ellis Island, circa 1917.
Courtesy of the National Park Service, Statue of Liberty National Monument, STLI 5052.

however. Later they would look back on their time on Ellis Island with fond memories. As Glenna Bigelow described it, on Ellis Island they were "cozy and comfortable . . . with good beds, plenty of heat, and unlimited hot baths."[52] They also had three square meals a day and clean uniforms. More importantly they were safe from gunfire, bombs, and mustard gas.

Later, just miles from the battlefront, the nurses soon experienced the reality of war. In France they lived in poorly insulated quarters heated by tiny stoves, washed with water from large gallon pitchers, and worked in makeshift hospitals surrounded by quagmires of mud, all the while aware of the distant sounds of "thunderous and continuous shelling."[53] As Chief Nurse Sarah Parsons of Base Hospital 6 later recalled, "Those first six months . . . who will ever forget them—dirt and smells and rats, scarcity of water and light."[54]

MILITARY EFFICIENCY

By the winter of 1918, the procedures for outfitting hundreds of nurses in a short time had been made quite efficient, and the nurses regularly made ferry trips to Manhattan for fittings of their uniforms and raincoats. Glenna Bigelow chronicled one episode in her diary, writing:

Tuesday, Feb 23—went en masse to the tailor's to be measured for uniforms . . . a hurried lunch and then to the rubber man for Sou'westers . . . and on to Cowards shoe store for boots.

The boot store was pandemonium, and it took more than two hours to convince anybody that we knew where we were going and what we wanted . . . as regards foot covering. As a matter of fact, we did not know either, so we took what was offered and straggled home in disorganized squads.[55]

The process was more organized than she thought, and later in the week, Glenna acknowledged that fact:

Friday our equipment arrived on the ferryboat, great packages and boxes from New York. We stood in line alphabetically to receive our consignment and marveled at the order and dispatch with which that great pile of things was dissipated. Every person's name was on exactly the right box, in exactly the right place, so that there was no confusion and presently we found ourselves back in our dormitory, staggering under our load of gifts.[56]

Sorting through their new uniforms and equipment was not the nurses' only pastime. The women spent a great deal of time getting to know each other, dancing to "the Victrola in Dormitory No. 2," practicing their French, celebrating birthdays, and attending Red Cross dances and movie nights. As Emma Weaver of Base Hospital 20 stated, "for the most part" the island was "permeated by a spirit of cheer."[57]

As the winter months dragged on and disturbing war news arrived from Europe, the emotional tone on Ellis Island turned more somber. Newly inducted nurses were now told to take out "war insurance policies" and write their last wills and testaments. Military drills became a daily ritual so that the nurses could "pivot and turn corners, keep in step, and march like soldiers."[58] Meanwhile, about five hundred Navy men were bivouacked on Island 1 in order to have them readily available should they be needed to sail at the last minute.[59] In addition, spies, enemy agents, and the officers and men of German merchant ships arrived to be imprisoned on the island. Indeed, Ellis Island was under "martial law; guards everywhere."[60] Recalling those days, Chief Nurse Edith Mury provided a succinct description, writing, "Between nurses 'parading in uniform' and 'interned Germans and imprisoned German agents under heavy guard,' the whole atmosphere was covered with 'a shadow of apprehension.'"[61]

That foreboding atmosphere clouded embarkations as well. Even on the brightest days, departures assumed a more solemn tone as the nurses began to understand the reality of what they would face in Europe. Glenna Bigelow described the scene from the perspective of a recruit awaiting her own sailing orders:

> The sky was blue, and the sun shone brightly on the little procession
> of 50 nurses, so dignified and smart in their dark blue uniforms.
> They emerged from their quarters, marched silently along the quay of
> Island #3, and over the bridge to the Chapel on Island #1, where we lost
> sight of them for a moment. Soon they came out and marched, two by
> two, toward the tender that was to take them out to their ship. . . . The
> silence was terrible; no fanfare of trumpets, no admiring friends,
> no flowers, only the grimness of parting.[62]

THE WAR DEPARTMENT REQUISITIONS ELLIS ISLAND HOSPITALS

With increasing numbers of injured soldiers returning from Europe, the US Army needed somewhere to put them before they were transferred to military hospitals closer to their homes. As a result, in late February 1918 the army requisitioned the Ellis Island hospitals for this purpose and ordered Margaret Daly and her staff to leave the General Hospital and report for assignment to Stapleton Marine Hospital on Staten Island.[63] Effective March 8, the army's administrative offices and surgeries took place in the Ellis Island General Hospital on Island 2, renamed Debarkation Hospital No. 1. In addition, the Contagious Disease Hospital buildings on Island 3 were designated as additional space for up to five hundred patients at a time.[64] The change required everything to move to the mainland: all nurse mobilization activities, soldiers and sailors who were already in recovery, and any "arriving immigrants requiring hospitalization."[65]

Not all Base Hospital nursing units left the island during the first week of March, however. Through late March and into April some Red Cross Army nurses remained on the island to care for soldiers returning from Europe, many of whom were transported back to the United States on the SS *Comfort*. Among the nurses left to receive them was Emma Weaver, a nurse from Base Hospital 20, who had arrived on Ellis Island only two weeks before the War Department commandeered the hospital buildings. Now Emma had orders to report to Chief Nurse Edith B. Irwin, who was for the short term in charge of the US Army Hospital.[66] According to Emma:

> March 1: Ellis Island was turned over as a receiving station for wounded soldiers coming from abroad. They [are] to be kept here temporarily until assigned to permanent hospitals. The nurses of Base Hospital #20 are put on duty temporarily while awaiting sailing orders.

> March 17: "Specialed" [sic] a case of diphtheria—a boy from Nebraska . . . died. I was given a dose of diphtheria antitoxin, which knocked me out completely. . . in bed all day Sunday. Tonight, a ship arrived bringing back 100 of our American boys—12 insane and 40 tuberculars; some wounded.[67]

Emma and her colleagues cared for those returning soldiers—some sick with infectious diseases like tuberculosis and diphtheria, others with war injuries or "shell shock"—until April 10, when other army nurses arrived with specific orders to staff Debarkation Hospital No. 1 and the members of Base Hospital 20 departed for overseas.[68]

Nurse Burnham with soldiers
on Ellis Island, circa 1917.
*Courtesy of the National Park Service, Statue
of Liberty National Monument, STLI 5052.*

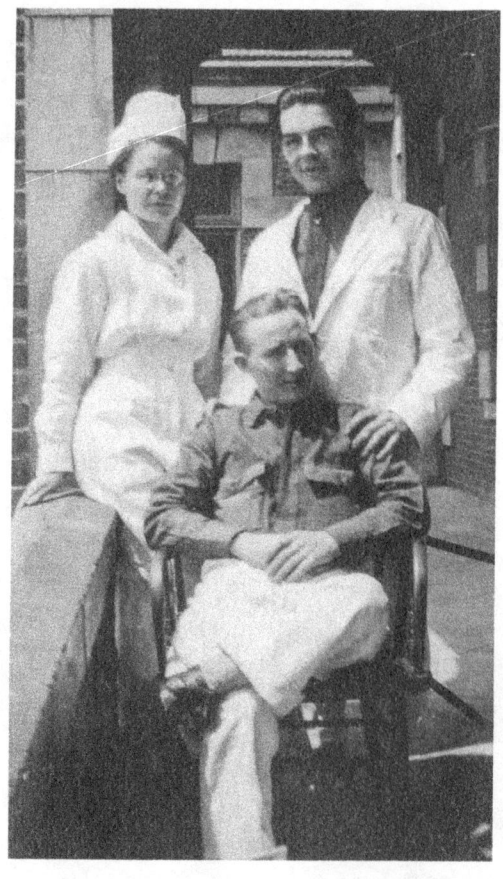

The newly arrived army nurses were soon busy. During the spring of 1918, Debarkation Hospital No. 1 admitted ten to twenty patients every day, all of them suffering from high fevers, coughs, and body aches.[69] First diagnosed with "three-day fever," these soldiers later would be classified as among the first wave of patients suffering from a virulent strain of influenza that had begun to circle the globe.[70]

The nurses soon fell ill with the 1918 flu as well. While most recovered, two of the army nurses assigned to Debarkation Hospital No. 1, Catherine Connolly and Mary J. Scheirer, died in the pandemic. Of the two, Catherine contracted the devastating virus first. She died on August 27, 1918, within eighteen hours of the onset of symptoms.[71] Mary Scheirer, a 1914 graduate of the Reading Hospital School of Nursing in Pennsylvania, also succumbed. She had volunteered to join the US Army Nurse Corps in April 1918 and was immediately sent to Debarkation Hospital No. 1 on Ellis Island to care for returning soldiers. In early autumn, with a third wave of influenza rampaging the island and the New York area, Mary contracted the lethal virus herself and died on October 5, 1918.[72]

RETURN OF THE USPHS STAFF AFTER THE WAR

Working through the remainder of the fall and into the winter and spring of 1919, the army nurses assigned to Debarkation Hospital No. 1 continued to care for returning soldiers as the United States demobilized its troops after the war ended on November 11, 1918. Finally, on June 30, 1919, the US Army formally evacuated Ellis Island, dispersing the soldiers to other military hospitals across the country and leaving only twenty-three immigrant patients in the island's hospital.[73]

That same day, having been ordered by the USPHS to return to Ellis Island, Margaret Daly left her post on Staten Island and reported for duty at the General Hospital (the newly vacated Debarkation Hospital No. 1). She took charge of five wards: two considered "general," one "venereal," and two "psychopathic."[74] She was ready—at least she thought she was until she entered the hospital. Looking around, Margaret gasped. The army had left the hospital in "frightful condition." The wards were a mess, remnants of dressings and used equipment were strewn everywhere. Windows and floors were covered in grime. The walls were marked and needed paint. Wasting no time, Margaret picked up a bucket and some cloths and turned to her staff. Together they would begin a thorough "cleaning crusade."[75]

With so much work to do, Margaret was relieved to hear that the nurses she had worked with at Stapleton Hospital, Margaret L. Burke, Helen Gennoy, Katherine O'Connell, and Sibyl Norris, would arrive in early July.[76] The days passed all too quickly. While Margaret and the newly arrived nurses were still painting the last of fifty-two beds, another wave of patients with influenza began to arrive "in droves," filling all available beds. Margaret recalled, "So crowded were we that we were obliged to turn the patients' dining rooms into wards. . . . Every nook and cranny was used for hospital purposes."[77] To make matters worse, a number of nurses came down with the flu themselves. Describing those days, Margaret later remarked, "For a time the situation seemed out of hand, but eventually difficulties were overcome, and we again resumed our normal routine."[78]

A normal routine was welcomed, as was an increase in numbers of immigrants arriving to the United States after the war. But that familiar rhythm was short-lived. In 1921, Congress passed the first of a series of restrictive immigration policies that would effectively end the era of mass immigration and permanently transform hospital activities on Ellis Island.

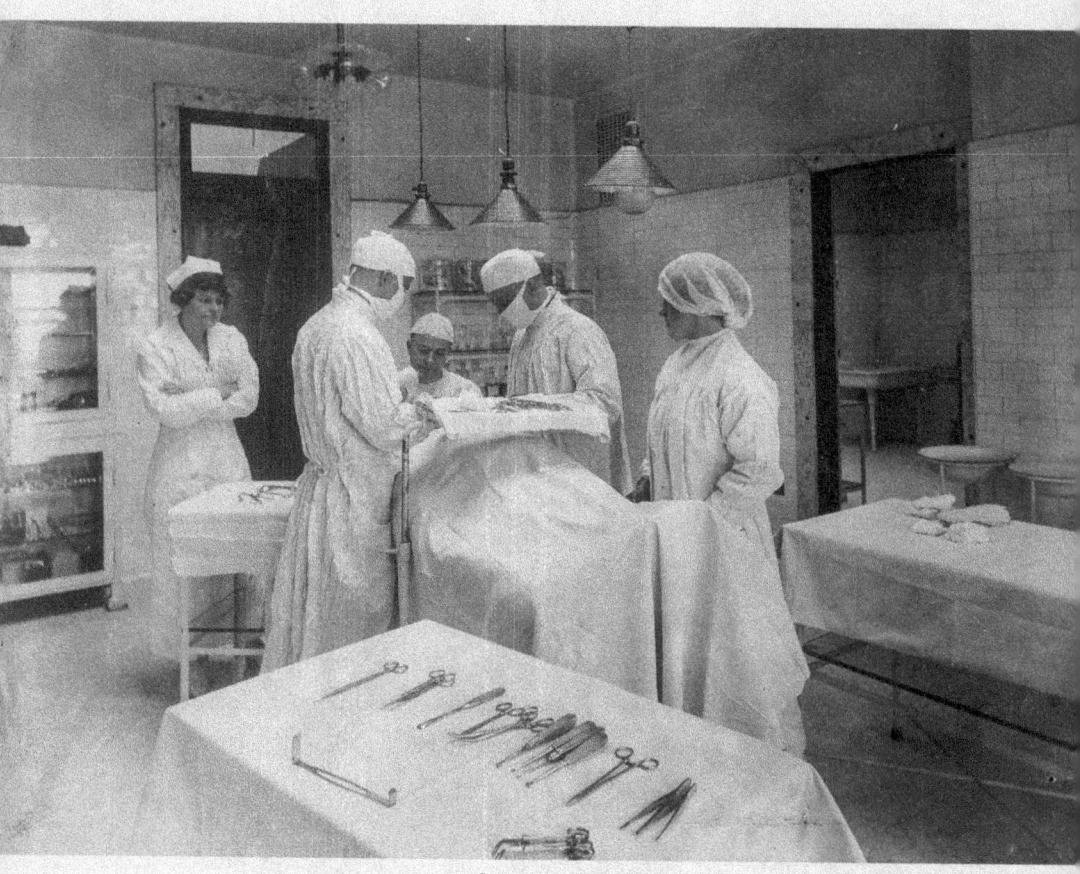

Surgery on Ellis Island.
Courtesy of the National Park Service, Statue of Liberty National Monument, STLI 24602.

CHAPTER 5

CHANGING RULES AND CHANGING ROLES 1920–1939

*Nurses are essential on account of the character of the patients handled
and the emergency nature of the work. This hospital is in reality a
communicable disease and evacuation hospital.*

J. W. KERR, ASSISTANT SURGEON GENERAL, ELLIS ISLAND[1]

C hief Nurse Margaret Daly walked into her office, sat down at her desk, and let out a long breath. She had just come up from Ward 2 of the General Hospital, where Josephine Friedman, a young ward maid who worked in the pediatric wards on Island 3, had been admitted overnight with acute abdominal pain, nausea, and a low-grade fever.[2] Though Margaret's nurses frequently dealt with emergencies, they found it upsetting to care for one of their own. Margaret had felt the nurses' tension levels rise when Josephine presented with right-sided abdominal pain—the hallmark of appendicitis. After she had assisted ward nurse Anna Cohen with Josephine's vital signs and initial assessment, Margaret had waited at the bedside until Chief Medical Officer W. C. Billings confirmed the diagnosis. Indeed, Josephine had appendicitis.

In the early 1920s, appendicitis carried a high risk of mortality regardless of surgical intervention, so Dr. Billings chose a more conservative approach. His treatment plan for the young ward maid included a liquid diet and complete bed rest "with an ice bag over the appendix, to be continued during the stage of severe pain."[3] Dr. Billings also wrote strict orders for close observation, and the nurses knew to alert him immediately if Josephine showed any signs of clinical deterioration, at which point an appendectomy would be performed.

With everyone somewhat settled, Margaret was back in her office, taking a short break before she inspected and prepared the operating room in the event Josephine needed surgery. She also had to call Ellen Cartledge, chief nurse of Island 3, to report on Josephine's status and ask if she needed another ward maid to fill in.[4]

Reaching for the telephone receiver, Margaret gazed outside. It was a beautiful day, and her third-floor window offered a clear view of the Contagious Disease Hospital with just the tiniest glimpse of Lady Liberty beyond. Letting her eyes wander across the waterway between the islands, Margaret once again found herself a bit startled to see that the walkway connecting Islands 2 and 3 was now completely enclosed—an upgrade the US Army had completed during their occupation of the hospital complex.[5]

The renovation was just another reminder of how much had changed on Ellis Island since the Great War. Even the hospital complex had a new official name and she occasionally had to remind herself to write "Marine Hospital No. 43" on her reports.[6] Despite how fervently she had "expressed the desire to return" to the chief nurse position on Ellis Island after being temporarily transferred to Stapleton Marine Hospital during the war, Margaret admitted that the nature of nursing work on Ellis Island had changed significantly, largely a result of the new federal immigration laws.[7] With the drastic reduction in immigrant arrivals in the early 1920s, Ellis Island nursing now involved "less immigration work" than it did "Marine Hospital work."[8] Servicemen and their beneficiaries had begun to account for a larger percentage of their patients.

Ellen's voice on the other end of the line pulled Margaret away from her thoughts. The two chief nurses scheduled a meeting for later that day, assuming they would have an update on Josephine's condition by that time. Margaret then set off toward the operating room just down the hall.[9]

SURGICAL NURSING ON ELLIS ISLAND

Located on the third floor, the operating room in the General Hospital had served as a prominent example of the state-of-the-art treatment offered on Ellis Island since the new building opened in 1902. Multiple skylights and large windows offered abundant natural lighting; white tile floors and walls made for easy cleaning; and a connected sterilization room, complete with an autoclave, ensured that surgical instruments were ready for use. The

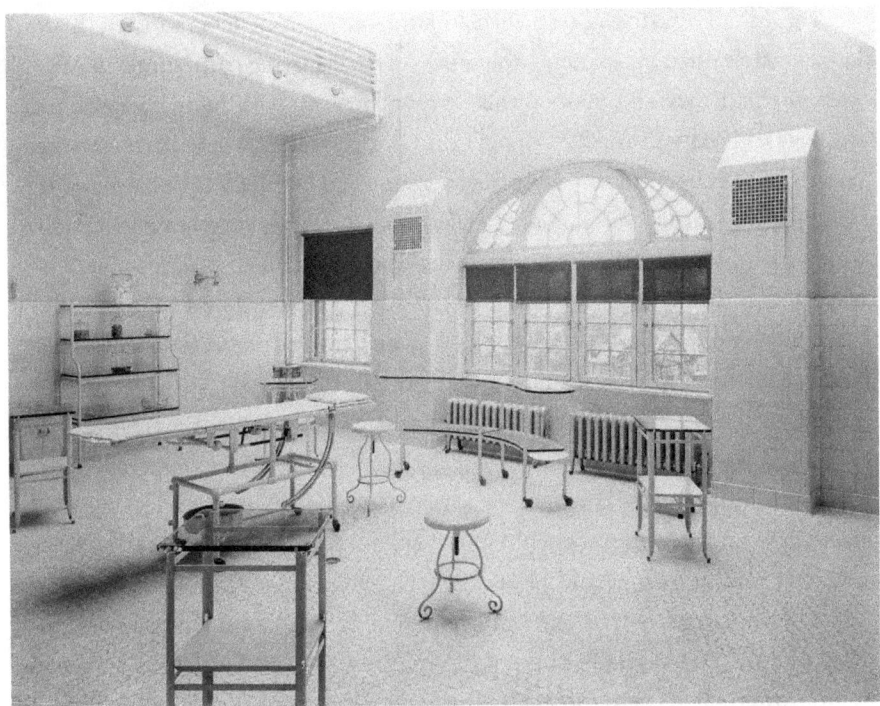

Empty third floor operating room in Ellis Island hospital, circa 1909.
Courtesy of the Library of Congress, Prints and Photographs Online Catalog.

adjacent "scrub-up room" was outfitted with contemporary surgical scrubbing equipment, including "nail brushes and orange sticks," as well as a basin of green soap with a "knee control" for hands-free operation.[10] Detailed USPHS protocols outlined the standards for cleaning the operating room, the operative supplies to be kept on hand, and the standards of conduct expected of all surgical staff.

The operating room on Ellis Island reflected not only the practical requirements of modern surgery but also the elite professional status of the surgeons themselves. Surgery had recently ascended to the top of the hierarchy of medical specialties. US Army surgeon John Shaw Billings felt the status was justified because "the most important improvements in practical medicine made in the United States" had been "chiefly in surgery."[11] Those improvements included the discovery of intraoperative anesthesia in the mid-nineteenth century and the application of the aseptic technique in the surgical theater a few decades later.[12]

The use of anesthesia transformed surgeons from butchers to artists. No longer constrained by a patient's tolerance for excruciating pain, surgeons could work meticulously and methodically, experimenting with more complex and invasive techniques to create opportunities for treatment where there had previously been none.[13] But surviving the operation and making a full recovery were two separate hurdles for patients to overcome. Surgical outcomes had actually worsened in the decades after anesthesia was introduced, primarily because of an increased incidence in postoperative infection and shock.[14] Not until the introduction of Joseph Lister's antiseptic principles and the subsequent reduction in infection rates did surgical mortality truly improve.[15]

Surgical innovation continued during and after World War I, shaped largely by the environment and experience of military physicians on the front lines. Wound infection rates skyrocketed when injured soldiers were left for days in muddy, rat-infested trenches. As a result, surgeons discovered the value of delaying wound closure and physically or chemically debriding diseased tissue.[16] New weapons of war, particularly exploding artillery shells, caused complex wounds and multiple penetrating traumas, forcing battlefield surgeons to improve their recognition and management of shock. The 1914 discovery of sodium citrate, a powerful anticoagulant, allowed blood to be stored in field hospitals and later transfused to soldiers suffering from hemorrhagic injuries.[17] Finally, the distinctive shrapnel injuries of World War I propelled surgical specialization. Shrapnel caused "very bad wounds" because it ripped, tore, and lacerated tissues, leading to vascular injuries, embedded foreign bodies, and extensive bone damage.[18] Thus, surgical specialties evolved as physicians developed expertise and skill in a specific operative process or organ system. For example, the increase in traumatic fractures and amputations fueled the rise of orthopedics, and the prevalence of extensive facial injuries pioneered the field of plastic surgery.[19]

Since the turn of the twentieth century, advancements in science, medicine, and surgery had altered the practice of surgical nursing, changing both the management of the operating room environment and the operative process itself. Almost every day, nurses had new responsibilities. They were required to apply principles of antisepsis in preparing the surgical theater and equipment; to supervise and manage operating room personnel; and to care for patients before, during, and after surgery.[20] According to a 1903 article in the *American*

Journal of Nursing, an efficient operating room nurse "must have the knowledge of how to make and keep things sterile, be familiar with surgical instruments and their particular uses, and have had a training which has fitted her to care intelligently for all the different kinds of operative cases."[21] Now, as surgical specialization grew after the war, nurses were also expected to learn a continuously expanding repertoire of operative techniques and how each one would affect their patients. By 1924 surgical nursing on Ellis Island had become so specialized that the USPHS hired a dedicated operating room nurse, Emma L. Colebourn.[22]

Approaching the operating suite, Margaret found Emma standing next to the autoclave, sterilizing the instruments needed for the day's scheduled surgeries. Initially the two women had distrusted one another, likely in response to Emma's additional role as acting assistant chief nurse of Island 2, reporting directly to Margaret. As Margaret recalled, when Emma had first arrived at Ellis Island, she "did not care for the Station and perhaps did not care for me either."[23] Fortunately, their animosity did not last long, and Margaret realized that Emma was a woman "of high type, very capable and efficient."[24] They soon became "very dear friends."[25] That camaraderie helped a great deal on busier days like today, when an emergency surgery or a lineup of multiple cases necessitated the rapid turnaround of surgical instruments and the operating room itself.

As soon as Margaret explained Josephine's condition, the two nurses fell into a comfortable and familiar professional rhythm as they worked to prepare the surgical suite. They knew the drill since the surgical service on Ellis Island averaged thirty to sixty operations each month.[26] The USPHS procedures dictated that "on the morning of the operation," the nurses must first wash the floors, wipe down the furniture, and resterilize the instruments, sutures, and linen.[27] So, while the two nurses conferred, Emma disinfected the surgical instruments, adding catgut and silkworm sutures to the next batch. They were "boiled in a 1% solution of sodium carbonate under live steam for 20 minutes."[28] She then sterilized all the enamelware, glassware, and rubber goods in the same manner. But she took extra care with the surgical knives and scissors, which were "sterilized in 95% carbolic for 20 minutes, then in alcohol for 10 minutes." These tools required extra attention to mitigate the increased risk of infection that occurred when objects penetrated the body.[29] Finished with this task, Emma placed the instruments on a wheeled surgical cart, covered the cart with a sterile towel, and moved it next to the operating room table.

While Emma attended to these preparations, Margaret focused on gathering the rest of the necessary supplies. She inventoried the sterile linens, counting the sponges, dressings, towels, and sheets. Then she ensured that enough gowns, rubber gloves, caps, and masks were available in the dressing room for the whole surgical team. If Josephine needed an appendectomy, Surgeon R. H. Heterick would lead that surgical team, consisting of a USPHS intern standing in as the surgical assistant and another as the anesthetist. Emma would "scrub in" as the sterile nurse, passing instruments to Dr. Heterick, while Margaret would serve as the "unsterile nurse," circulating the room as necessary.[30] USPHS policy mandated that all operating room staff wear surgical gowns and caps; however, the use of face masks was required only in "abdominal, bone and joint cases."[31]

Operating room procedures also specified which supplies had to be on hand in the event of any surgical emergencies, including anesthesia overdoses and hypovolemic shock. The physicians on Ellis Island delivered anesthesia to the patient by the open drop method, which could prove deadly if the anesthetist overzealously administered the ether. Although Margaret trusted all of the USPHS surgeons implicitly, she made sure to place a "hypodermic syringe containing 1/30 gr. Strychnine sulphate for use in emergency" right next to the fresh can of ether she set out for the anesthetist.[32] That way, if a patient fell into "anesthesia narcosis," the surgeon could immediately administer the drug, noted for its "great value" as a cardiac and respiratory stimulant.[33] Margaret also made sure the "complete salvarsan apparatus" for giving intravenous (IV) solutions had been sterilized within the last week, checking that a "good supply of normal salt solution" was on hand in case the surgeon needed to administer IV fluids to the patient during the operation.[34]

Fortunately, Josephine did not require the emergency surgery for which Margaret and Emma had prepared. Instead, her appendicitis resolved itself with symptom management and close observation. Later Josephine recalled the quality of care she received, saying, "They treated me royally . . . just like one of the first-class patients that came in."[35]

While the nurses undoubtedly gave Josephine special attention because they wanted to help a fellow staff member, they likely had the extra time to do so, given the reduced number of patients in the hospital. Recent changes to the federal immigration policy had already begun to impact medical and nursing services on the island.

NEW IMMIGRATION LAWS AND THE END OF MASS IMMIGRATION

Between the passage of the Immigration Act of 1891 and the United States' entrance into World War I in 1917, Congress had approved several increasingly restrictive immigration laws. Rather than restricting the total number of new arrivals, the immigration laws prior to the 1920s focused on qualitative control by identifying specific types of undesirable conditions that immigrants might manifest that would disqualify them from entering the United States and mandate their immediate deportation. The list of excludable conditions grew to include proscribed moral and social behaviors, such as those attributable to anarchists, prostitutes, and criminals, as well as a broader range of medical diagnoses, including "imbeciles, feeble-minded persons, [and] epileptics."[36] The Immigration Act of 1917 identified a record thirty-three categories for mandatory exclusion and deportation of immigrants, few of which posed any danger of contagion. A literacy test was added to the medical inspection process. The new policies contrasted sharply with the first federal immigration law, written to balance immigrants' freedoms to pursue opportunity in the United States with the government's responsibility to protect its citizens from epidemic disease. Now, rather than preventing the introduction of dangerous or contagious illness, these newer and more restrictive laws reflected nativist fears surrounding a growing threat of political radicalism and the weakening of "American stock."[37]

Anti-immigrant sentiments were sparked nationwide both during and after World War I. The rush of war refugees to America during the immediate postwar period, driven by political and economic unrest across the European continent, added fuel to the fire. Most of these immigrants hailed from southern and eastern Europe, and many Americans viewed them as poor, uneducated, and more difficult to assimilate than their western European counterparts. Considered both an economic and cultural threat to Anglo-Saxon Americans, the southern and eastern Europeans were described by anti-immigrant activists as "the dependents, the human wreckage of the war."[38] As cities across the United States faced industrial uncertainty, rising unemployment, and housing shortages in the aftermath of World War I, pressure mounted for Congress to take extreme action regarding immigration. Congress responded by passing the most restrictive legislation to date.

Initially written as a temporary measure, the 1921 Emergency Quota Law ushered in the quantitative era of immigration policy. The law placed a numerical cap on the total number of immigrants allowed to enter the United States each year, broken down by country of origin, with approximately 350,000 total visas available to new immigrants. Using racial and ethnic population totals from the 1910 census, the quota formula established that no more than 3 percent of any nationality would be permitted each year.[39] Only 20 percent of that annual allowance would be entitled to enter the United States each month. Moreover, immigrants would still be required to pass a medical inspection and a hearing with the Board of Special Inquiry upon their arrival. Those who failed were sent to increasingly crowded detention rooms where contagious disease ran rampant.[40]

CONTAGIOUS DISEASES AMONG DETAINEES

Prior to the discovery and widespread deployment of vaccines and antibiotics in the mid-twentieth century, infectious disease was a leading cause of death throughout the world. In the early twentieth century, improved sanitation, hygiene, and knowledge of how diseases spread helped to reduce overall mortality, but tens of thousands of US citizens still died each year of contagious illness. Young children suffered higher mortality rates than adults.

In the overcrowded detention quarters on Ellis Island, infectious disease spread quickly and quietly among the anxious new arrivals awaiting their hearing with the Board of Special Inquiry. Results were sometimes fatal, reflecting the worst rather than the typical immigrant experiences on Ellis Island. For two immigrants, a confluence of situational circumstances—the restrictive new quota laws, the sociopolitical pressure to scrutinize new arrivals more carefully, the USPHS staffing challenges, the idiosyncrasies in the categorization of certain medical conditions, and the limits of contemporary medical science—ultimately ended in tragedy. Ormond Joseph McDermott and Ruth Grahn were two of the thirty-five hundred patients who died in the Ellis Island hospitals despite the excellent nursing care they received.

ORMOND JOSEPH MCDERMOTT AND SCARLET FEVER NURSING

On February 16, 1921, Ormond Joseph McDermott, a nineteen-year-old immigrant from Sydney, Australia, arrived in New York Harbor on the steamship *Wandilla*. The eldest of nine children, "Little O. J." had sailed to the United States after securing a visa to complete a one-year apprenticeship at the Studebaker Car Company in South Bend, Indiana.[41] During his immigration processing on Ellis Island, officials questioned Ormond's claim that he had earned his passage as a working member of the ship's crew. His appearance hadn't helped. Ormond had dressed in his best suit, tie, cuffed shirt, and overcoat in the manner that many immigrants knew could help them get into the country. However, the officials didn't think Ormond's attire fit the description of a typical "workaway" seaman.[42] Making matters worse, Ormond inadvertently had left his passport and proof of temporary worker status in his cabin aboard the *Wandilla*. Ellis Island officials, refusing to allow the young man to retrieve his paperwork, held him in the detention rooms on Island 1 while they investigated his immigration status.

Awaiting his hearing, Ormond spent the next nine days in crowded, close quarters with other immigrants, some sick; some well. Aware of the "increased prevalence of communicable diseases and decreased vitality among war populations," the USPHS physicians had initiated daily medical rounds in the detention areas to identify anyone in need of medical attention.[43] During evening rounds on February 25, 1921, the USPHS staff discovered that Ormond had a fever, sore throat, and "general erythematous rash" over his chest and abdomen. Suspecting that Ormond might have scarlet fever, the physicians immediately sent him to Isolation Ward 4 in the Contagious Disease Hospital.[44]

At nineteen years old, Ormond had not been part of the mandatory temperature screening performed twice daily for all young children in the detention rooms; no doubt his fever and early symptoms had gone unnoticed for days. Now, however, under the care of Nurse Neilson, he was observed closely. Having received the "rather acutely ill" young man to her ward in the Contagious Disease Hospital, Nurse C. Nielson followed Dr. Richeson's orders to "paint [the patient's] throat with argyrol 20% stat."[45] Overnight, she also gave Ormond aspirin every four hours and administered the liquid diet that had been prescribed.

Within twenty-four hours, Dr. Richeson determined that McDermott's rash appeared "very much like scarlet fever" and transferred him to Ward 13, where he received more specialized, disease-specific treatment.[46] Both Nurse Nielson and Dr. Richeson were concerned. While death was "rare in cases that receive proper care and attention," mild cases of scarlet fever could quickly progress to severe disease as the *Streptococcus pyogenes* bacteria spread to other parts of the body, causing complications of the heart, lungs, kidneys, and nervous system.[47] Ormond's transfer to Ward 13 was definitely warranted.

Designated for active cases of diphtheria, mumps, chickenpox, and scarlet fever, Ward 13 contained twenty beds "arranged in thirteen cubicles or small rooms" to maintain isolation between patients and reduce the chance of cross infection.[48] There, Ormond would receive expert, intensive care from USPHS nursing staff who understood the gravity of his condition and could recognize changes that indicated a need for further medical intervention.

As soon as Ormond arrived on the ward on February 26, 1921, acting assistant surgeon W. H. Turner took cultures of McDermott's nose and throat and sent those to the lab to rule out the possibility of diphtheria or tuberculosis.[49] In the decade since the Contagious Disease Hospital first opened, significant advancements had been made in the science of bacteriology and laboratory diagnostics; as a result, the USPHS medical staff increasingly utilized routine cultures and blood tests to diagnose and monitor contagious illness.[50] (Though the causative bacteria for scarlet fever would not be identified until 1924, culture results would definitively rule out other diseases like diphtheria or tuberculosis.) Dr. Turner also prescribed a liquid diet, Brown's mixture for any cough, and a frequent gargle of Dobell's solution—an antiseptic mixture of carbolic acid, sodium bicarbonate, and sodium borate intended to neutralize the bacteria in Ormond's throat and prevent the infection from spreading to the rest of his body.

Following Dr. Turner's orders meticulously, nurses Lucy Simpson and Edna Miller cared for Ormond throughout his stay in Ward 3. They bathed Ormond daily, checked his vital signs every four hours, gave him milk and other liquids for nutrition and hydration, and washed his mouth with Dobell's solution. They also kept detailed nurses' notes, documenting that Ormond spent his first two days quietly, slept well, and did not have much of a cough.[51]

On the evening of February 28, however, Nurse Lucy Simpson noted that Ormond's condition was beginning to deteriorate rapidly as evidenced by his increased restlessness during the night and his several attempts to get out of bed.[52] That night Lucy spent the majority of her shift at Ormond's bedside, closely monitoring him. Finally, in the early morning of March 1, Lucy telephoned Dr.

Turner when her patient's temperature, pulse, and respiratory rate were all well outside the normal range.

By this time, Ormond was critically ill, likely septic and suffering cardiac and pulmonary complications as the infection spread throughout his body. In fact, Dr. Turner noted that Ormond had become "rather toxic"; he would not survive another twenty-four hours.[53] Indeed, Ormond's temperature soared above 105 degrees Fahrenheit, and his heart and respiratory rates climbed along with it.[54] His rapid pulse had become weak and thready and his breath sounds diminished as his heart failed and fluid accumulated in his lungs.

Lucy and the other nurses continued to closely observe their patient, monitoring his restlessness, and attempting to comfort him through the worst of his symptoms. They gave him baths in an attempt to reduce his high fever, offered him milk and water to keep him hydrated, and repeatedly cleaned his throat with the prescribed argyrol and Dobell's solution. As Ormond's condition worsened, his physician prescribed Dover's powder, an opium-based analgesic to induce rest, and digitalis to reduce his heart rate and improve his circulation.[55] Nothing worked. By 11:30 p.m., Lucy found her patient "covered with cold perspiration" and noted that his arms were "cold to [the] elbows"; his pulse was "very weak."[56] Within the hour, Ormond was dead.[57]

Per the USPHS policy for care of deceased patients, Lucy called Dr. Turner, the medical officer in charge, who officially pronounced Ormond dead at 12:25 a.m. on March 2, 1921, and left the room. Lucy then wrapped Ormond's body "in a sheet wrung out of disinfectant solution" and tied an identification tag to the sheet before requesting the body be transferred to the morgue.[58] Ormond McDermott's body was then placed in a lead-lined coffin for steamship transport back to his family in Sydney, along with his personal effects. Listed among his clothes, shoes, and hat was the British passport that could have prevented Ormond's detention in the first place.[59]

RUTH GRAHN AND OBSTETRIC CARE ON ELLIS ISLAND

On December 21, 1923, Ruth Grahn, an unmarried, twenty-eight-year-old pregnant woman from Sweden, arrived in New York Harbor on the steamship *Kungsholm*. She too would be the victim of an unfortunate illness suffered during her detention on Ellis Island. Discovering "conclusive clinical evidence" of Ruth's pregnancy during the inspection process, a USPHS physician marked her condition on the medical certificate form in accordance with the regulations.[60] Pregnancy was categorized as a Class B condition, a "defect or disease" that could "affect the ability of the alien for self-maintenance."[61] Ruth's Class B medical certificate required her to go in front of the Board of Special Inquiry. During her hearing, Ruth stated that she was "in good health . . . about seven months pregnant but able to travel."[62] The board decided that she should be deported, declaring her "likely to become a public charge" because of her unmarried status.[63] Using her right to an appeal, Ruth challenged the board's decision and was "placed in detention to await the ruling by Washington."[64]

Ruth Grahn spent the next eleven days in the women's detention quarters on Island 1, complaining of cold, drafty rooms and an inability to stay warm "no matter how much clothes she put on."[65] A few days later, when Ruth's brother visited her, he immediately realized she was suffering from "a very severe cold."[66] Over the next week, Ruth developed a fever and "pain in her left chest," at which time her condition was reported to the USPHS officials.[67] On January 1, 1924, Ruth was admitted to Ward 3 of the Ellis Island General Hospital with a diagnosis of acute pleurisy, an inflammation of the lining of the lungs.[68]

Clearly Ruth needed nursing care. For the next ten days the Ellis Island nurses provided her "ordinary treatment" for pleurisy since she showed "no signs of impending labor."[69] Treating her fever and acute chest pain took priority. After placing her on bed rest, the nurses gave Ruth a bath to reduce her fever. Then they applied four-inch strips of adhesive plaster "as tightly as possible from the middle of the chest in front," around Ruth's left side, to the center of her back.[70] The tight bandage restricted the movement of Ruth's chest wall, thus reducing her pain. The nurses also applied cold compresses to her affected chest area and monitored her carefully.

Within several days, under the "excellent care and treatment" of the nursing staff, Ruth recovered—at least enough to be discharged from the hospital in accordance with the USPHS policies.[71] On January 10, Ruth was sent back to the detention area on Island 1 to wait for deportation. By this time, her appeal had been denied and the Board of Special Inquiry ordered her deportation on a ship sailing for Sweden on January 15. For the interim days before she was to sail, Ruth waited in the women's detention rooms, her only contact with the USPHS physicians occurring during their twice daily rounds. There she remained until she went into labor on January 14.

Immigrant births had been a regular occurrence on Ellis Island since the original forty-bed hospital opened in 1892. The USPHS nurses and physicians were well-prepared to handle obstetric cases despite the unique circumstances surrounding maternity care on the island. Hospital personnel could not predict when and how many pregnant immigrants would arrive or whether the expectant mothers would go into labor. Sometimes weeks passed without a single birth on Ellis Island, and sometimes multiple births occurred in a single night.[72] Moreover, given the lack of guaranteed citizenship for babies born on Ellis Island, many expectant mothers concealed their pregnancies or waited as long as possible before telling anyone that they were in labor.[73] In fact, as Chief Nurse Margaret Daly recalled, these mothers "were so anxious to be admitted [to the country] that they would stand in line until the baby would come right there."[74] As a result, many more births "occurred on the way to wards" than ever happened in the operating or delivery rooms.[75] This phenomenon prompted the Ellis Island nurses to create a portable obstetric pack containing sterile linens and other necessary supplies that could be used for emergency deliveries.[76] So, on January 14, when Ruth Grahn complained of labor pains, the USPHS surgeon Mary T. Mernin was "prepared to deliver her [right] there if necessary."[77] After an hour of close observation, however, Dr. Mernin determined that Ruth could be safely moved to the operating room in the General Hospital.

Ruth gave birth to a son at 4:30 p.m. that same day—the delivery described as "perfectly normal." An hour later, she was moved to the obstetric ward.[78] While the delivery may have been normal, Ruth's condition was not. During the admission examination, the USPHS surgeon H. M. Byington noted that Ruth was seriously ill, clearly showing signs of worsening pneumonia. She appeared pale and weak and had an elevated pulse rate as well as a "loose cough with blood-tinged sputum."[79] Recognizing her fragile state, Dr. Byington ordered "one to one" nursing care, worried that "the strain of childbirth" had likely exhausted much of Ruth's strength and "lowered her resisting power to pneumonia."[80] Dr. Byington had cause for worry. At the time, the United States had one of the highest maternal mortality rates in the world. Moreover, data from the 1918 influenza pandemic indicated that nearly 50 percent of postpartum women suffering from pneumonia died.[81] Ruth's case fit those criteria.

Unfortunately, even with intensive nursing care and advanced medical treatment, Ruth's condition became critical; she died at 6:22 p.m. on January 17,

1924. The baby no doubt was given to her family.[82] After a thorough investigation into the case, Surgeon General Hugh S. Cumming found no evidence of neglect or medical mismanagement and extended "a spirit of empathy and humanity" to Ruth Grahn's family from the medical and nursing corps on Ellis Island after her passing.[83] Her death, however, did not change the USPHS policies prohibiting unmarried pregnant women from entering the country. In fact, that same year, Congress passed the National Origins Act, setting additional limits on who could enter the United States.

THE 1924 NATIONAL ORIGINS ACT

The 1924 National Origins Act marked the official end of mass immigration to the United States. Advocating that "America must be kept American" (meaning, of course, that White Anglo-Saxon people maintain their majority), President Calvin Coolidge supported further restrictions on immigration, referring to the "present economic and social conditions" as the cause of the limitations.[84] Whatever his true motivation, the president passed the new law that allowed just 2 percent of the total population of each nationality to emigrate, reducing the annual total of available visas to 167,677.[85] Quota calculations were also reconfigured using population data from the 1890 census, which heavily favored immigrants from northern and western Europe and altogether excluded those from Asia. The new law led to an immediate and long-lasting reduction in the volume of immigrant arrivals being processed through the Ellis Island Station each year. Between 1924 and 1940, immigration through the Port of New York fell by nearly 90 percent.[86]

While each change in the immigration policy had caused some alteration to the USPHS procedures on Ellis Island, none had a more sweeping impact than the Immigration Act of 1924. In addition to severe numerical restrictions, the law also introduced the consular control system, which required that immigrants apply for a visa and undergo a medical inspection at the consulate in their home country *before* boarding a steamship. Though immigrants still passed through Line inspections on Ellis Island when they arrived in the Port of New York, the number of unexpected medical certificates leading to rejection and deportation decreased. Many USPHS and Immigration Department staff found the change to be a more humane process than the previous one. Describing the old method as a "gross injustice," Commissioner of Immigration Frederick A. Wallace noted that "examination on the other side is ten thousand times better than rejection on this side."[87]

As fewer immigrants were processed through Ellis Island, the number of immigrant patients in the hospitals also decreased. Admissions still occurred, mostly because the reduced volume of daily arrivals allowed for a new "intensive" method of examination by the USPHS physicians. They looked for anything that may have been missed during the consulate medical inspection and for any new medical issues that may have arisen during the weeks-long interval between the consulate inspection and the arrival on Ellis Island.[88] For this reason, "a certain amount of hospitalization" could always be anticipated to "take care of immigrants taken sick during their passage."[89] Nonetheless, as the number of immigrant admissions continued to decline, overcrowded local marine hospitals began to divert coastguardsmen, merchant seamen, and their beneficiaries to Ellis Island for treatment.

At the same time, Ellis Island experienced a marked increase in the number of "warrant cases"—immigrants who had already been admitted to the United

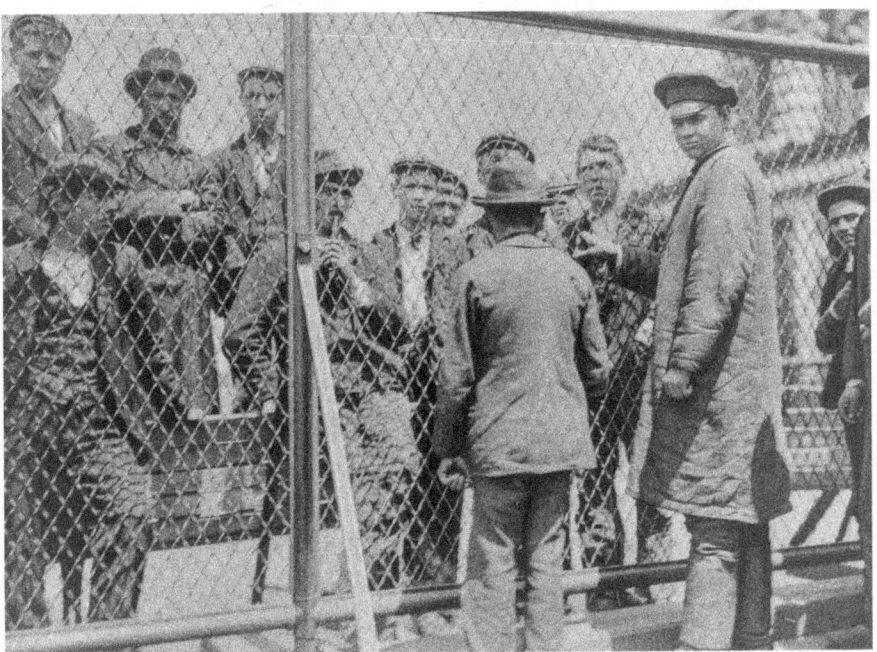

Detention pen on the roof of the Ellis Island Main Building, circa 1902–1910.
Courtesy of the Library of Congress, Prints and Photographs Online Catalog.

States but were under suspicion for violation of the federal immigration and deportation law. If a recently admitted immigrant fell into any of the excludable classes within five years of their arrival, they qualified for deportation. In these situations, the secretary of labor would issue a warrant and immigration officials would apprehend the immigrant in question and detain them in the nearest immigration station until their hearing before the local immigration board. The board would decide to either send the immigrant back into the United States or deport them to their country of origin. Beginning with the first "Red Scare" in the summer of 1919, the incidence of warrant detentions at Ellis Island rose so sharply that Immigration Commissioner Frederick C. Howe despaired, "I have become a jailer."[90]

Throughout the 1920s and 1930s, warrant cases continued to crowd the detention rooms on Island 1, with nearly three hundred thousand immigrants apprehended and sent to Ellis Island during that time.[91] A 1934 federal report concluded that the biggest problem on the island was "not that of the immigrant but that of the outgoing alien. . . . Sometimes they wait for long periods of time."[92] Every person with a warrant underwent a medical examination by the USPHS officials "for the purpose of finding those aliens afflicted with mental and contagious disease" and to find any immigrants "afflicted with medical and surgical conditions" that needed "hospital treatment."[93]

All that took time. Making matters worse, persistent staffing challenges for both the USPHS and the US Immigration Service contributed to bottlenecks in examining and processing the immigrant arrivals. This was especially problematic at the beginning of each month, a consequence of the language of the new quota laws. Working to avoid financial penalties for exceeding the 20 percent cap on each country's total number of immigrants allowed each month, transportation companies tried to "land their passengers as near the first of the month as possible" to avoid the possibility of their passengers arriving "in excess of the quota."[94] This surge of steamship arrivals meant that the bulk of immigrant examination work occurred during the first few days of the month, leaving the USPHS "seriously understaffed" and struggling to complete more intensive medical inspections.[95] Immigration officials also struggled to keep up, leading to delays in processing times with the Board of Special Inquiry. Detention rooms on Island 1 became increasingly congested as both new arrivals and warrant cases waited for their immigration hearing to be scheduled. These processing delays, which sometimes lasted for weeks, led British ambassador to the United States Sir Auckland Geddes to remark that "the very heart of the tragedy of Ellis Island is in the room of the temporarily detained."[96]

For Ellis Island nurses, these changes in the federal immigration policy and the USPHS procedures fundamentally altered the nature of their work as they addressed the various needs of the different patient populations admitted to the hospital. Many of the warrant immigrant cases were apprehended on suspicion of mental illness or another mandatory excludable medical condition, thus increasing the numbers of psychiatric patients needing hospitalization. Additionally, service members who transferred to Ellis Island from the local marine hospitals typically suffered from chronic conditions like mental illness or tuberculosis and needed extended courses of treatment.

PSYCHIATRIC NURSING ON ELLIS ISLAND

Throughout the 1920s and 1930s, nurses stationed at Ellis Island cared for increasing numbers of patients diagnosed with psychiatric conditions. Psychiatric nursing on the island had always been needed. The immigrants' long and difficult journey across the Atlantic, often experienced in cramped steerage-class conditions, induced or exacerbated their mental illness, causing some immigrants to arrive in mental health crises. Federal immigration policy also mandated that the USPHS identify and detain all "insane persons" until they could be deported to their country of origin.[97] Thus, in the decades after World War I, the changing sociopolitical context and different patient populations on Ellis Island, coupled with the evolution of medical understanding and the new approaches to neuropsychiatric treatment, meant the nurses saw a significant increase in the number of psychiatric cases under their observation and treatment at Marine Hospital No. 43.

PSYCHIATRIC CARE FOR IMMIGRANTS

Immigration law had always been clear and unyielding: psychiatric disorders were Class A conditions and immigrants thus certified would be "excluded from admission into the United States."[98] The earliest immigration restrictions focused on "insanity" and "idiocy"—each with very explicit medical definitions—but the number of prohibited medical conditions related to mental health broadened with each new federal policy. In 1907 "imbeciles," "feebleminded persons," those with a history of psychiatric issues, or anyone deemed "mentally defective" were added to the list of restricted classes; the Immigration Act of 1917 expanded the Class A designation even further to include "persons of constitutional psychopathic inferiority."[99]

The language used in the newer laws reflected the rising popularity of the eugenics movement within popular culture and the medical community. In broad terms, the goal of eugenics was to perfect the physical, mental, and moral health of society through improved human heredity. At the time, almost anything was classified as a hereditary trait, not just physical characteristics. Eugenic supporters considered poverty, criminal or immoral behavior, and susceptibility to disease to also be genetic defects. The practical application of eugenics meant that procreation was encouraged among "racially fitter stocks"— Anglo-Saxons with light skin, hair, and eyes—and actively discouraged or prevented among individuals deemed "obviously and grossly unfit."[100] Before and after World War I, anti-immigrant groups promoted baseless theories about the supposed mental inferiority and hereditary weakness of newer immigrants and used modern eugenic philosophy to strengthen those claims.

A number of immigration officials and USPHS surgeons either had ties to the eugenics movement or clearly agreed with eugenic theories. In 1912 Immigration Commissioner William Williams asserted that "mentally defective immigrants"—whom he referred to as "lumps of poisonous leaven"—were more dangerous and of "vastly greater concern" than those with infectious diseases.[101] In response, the mental examinations of immigrant arrivals became much more extensive.[102] USPHS physicians were instructed to make every effort "to detect signs and symptoms of mental disease and defect."[103] Medical inspection handbooks explicitly detailed every potential symptom and physical manifestation of certain psychiatric disorders, directing that any abnormality "no matter how trivial" was sufficient cause for a more thorough examination.[104] In addition to an extensive physical examination, the secondary inspection incorporated a mental fitness screening that initially included a racially biased personality test but eventually changed to block puzzles that were thought to reduce the impact of language differences and any lack of education on the test results.[105]

Even though immigrants with Class A psychiatric medical certificates were summarily excluded from admission to the United States, they needed a "suitable place" where they could be safely kept until officials could secure their return

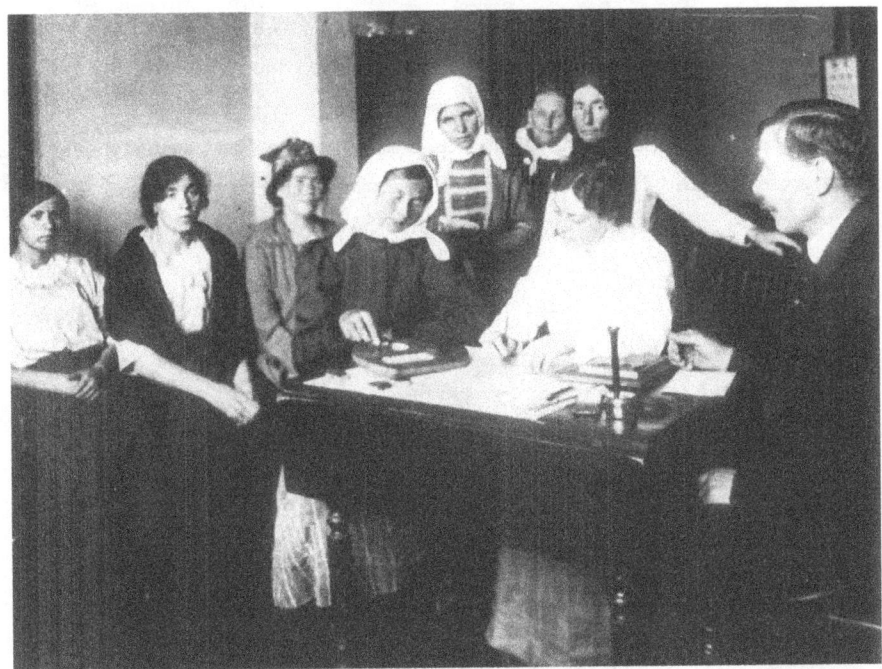

USPHS examiners perform mental testing of a female immigrant, circa 1920.
Courtesy of the National Archives at College Park, Still Pictures, 90-G-125-20.

transportation.[106] However, the original Ellis Island General Hospital did not include facilities specially tailored for the observation and care of immigrants suffering from acute psychiatric conditions. This design was an unfortunate oversight. Physicians acknowledged that admitting psychiatric patients to the General Hospital was "undesirable" because they would not receive the necessary care. The hospital's open ward design and busy nursing staff meant that psychiatric patients couldn't be monitored as closely or as carefully as needed during the acute phase of their illness, putting them and the USPHS staff in danger.[107] After two psychiatric patients died in 1906, Immigration Commissioner Robert Watchorn requested special facilities for this patient category, arguing that if Ellis Island "had proper accommodation neither of these suicides would have been possible."[108]

In November 1907 a new hospital building known as the "Psychopathic Pavilion" opened to immigrant patients. The two-story structure was erected off the connecting corridor between the General Hospital and the hospital outbuilding on Island 2. Each story contained a ten-bed ward, bathrooms, and several padded isolation rooms for "disturbed cases."[109] The design features of the building itself supported the patients' confinement, including locked doors and wire frames on every window that were to be "kept closed and securely locked."[110] On the west side of the building, a small, fully enclosed patio provided ambulatory patients with access to sunlight and fresh air while keeping them confined.

Nursing care for immigrants admitted to the psychiatric wards focused primarily on their safety. The smaller ward design (ten beds per ward rather than twenty) meant the nurses could closely observe their patients and intervene as

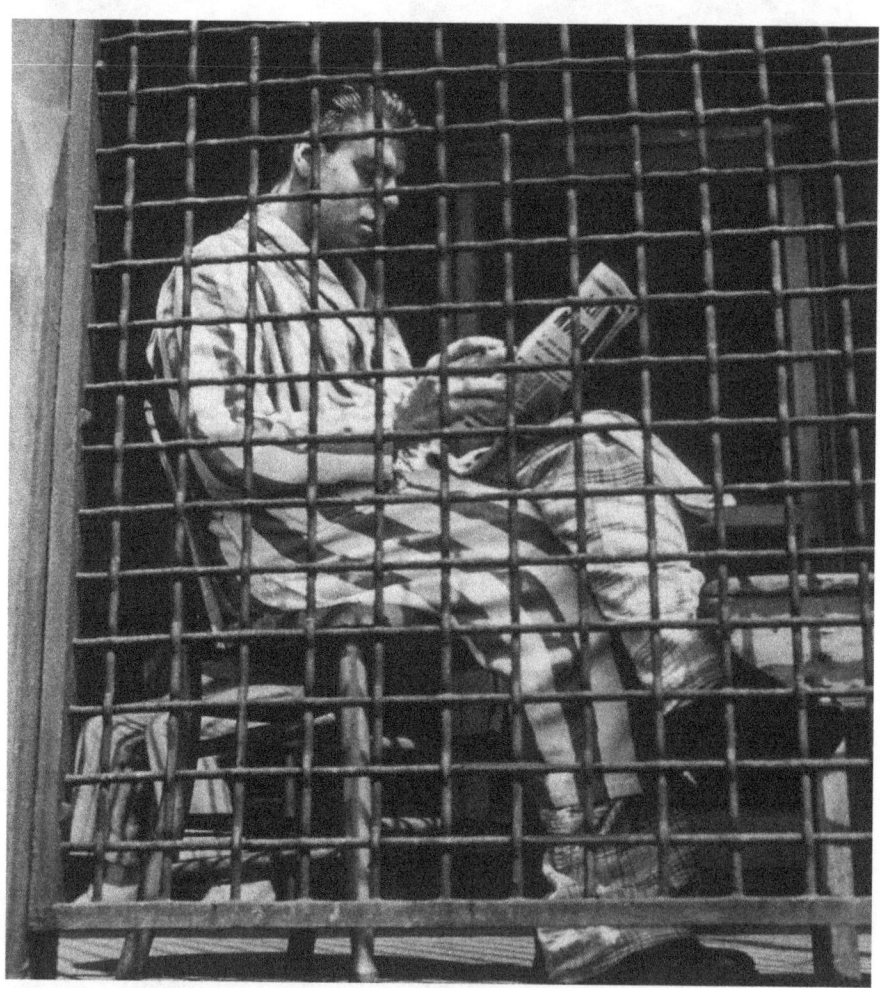

Detained patient in the enclosed porch of the men's psychiatric ward, circa 1930.
Courtesy of the National Library of Medicine Digital Collections.

soon as they demonstrated worsening symptoms. Driven by the custodial care and moral therapy approach to mental illness, the USPHS policies mandated that nurses isolate and detain patients in psychiatric distress while offering them compassionate support for their daily needs. Hospital stays were short, and the hospital staff offered little therapeutic treatment before these patients were deported. However, the nurses ensured the safety of their patients by minimizing the risks in the ward environment, provided good nutrition and encouraged their patients to eat, enforced structure through their daily routines, and gave

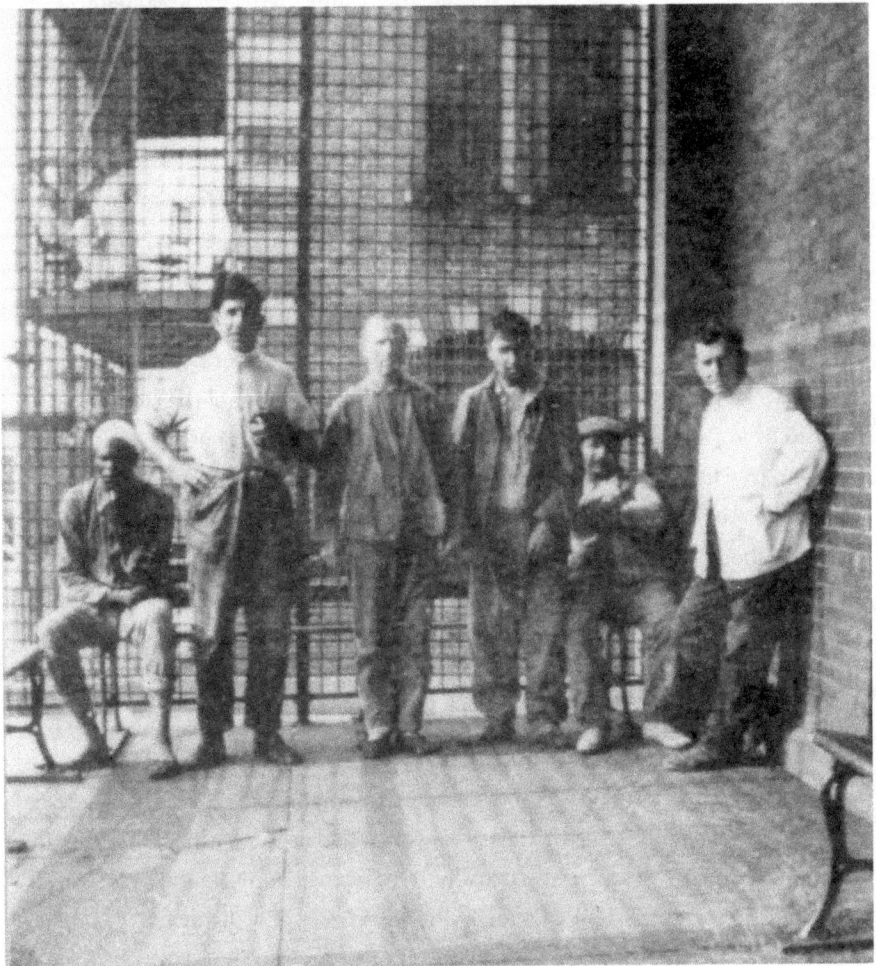

Ellis Island patients enjoying fresh air therapy on the enclosed porch of the men's psychiatric ward, circa 1930–1943.
Courtesy of the National Archives at College Park, Still Pictures, 90-G-125-53-3.

them opportunities for light exercise. The nurses ensured the doors to the unit remained locked and kept the keys with them at all times. In addition to following standard admission procedures, the nurses searched every psychiatric patient for any items that could be used to "do harm to themselves or others, such as knives," which they promptly turned over to the island registrar.[111] A nurse and ward maid at all times supervised the patients as they ate their provided meals three times daily on the ward. They approved only the use of spoons as a feeding utensil.[112] The nurses also provided their patients with moderate exercise, but it was "limited to walking about the wards" and pacing on the enclosed patio at the end of the pavilion.[113]

For the nurses assigned to psychiatric duty, Chief Nurse Margaret Daly gave explicit instructions: remain vigilant and always abide by the USPHS regulations for conduct on the wards. Margaret had reason for the strict orders, as she had once been threatened by a psychiatric patient while she performed her daily rounds of the General Hospital. That particular day, after discovering an orderly had not reported for his shift, Margaret told the head attendant to supervise breakfast for the ambulatory patients. She turned her back to answer the telephone and suddenly "felt something cold" pressed against the back of her neck while a large male patient demanded the ward keys.[114] Luckily, a member of the cleaning staff walked by and Margaret used the distraction to push the patient against the wall and separate herself; the patient, realizing he'd lost his opportunity, walked away to join the others for breakfast. The incident left her "frightened" and "trembling all over," though she had never before been fearful of psychiatric patients.[115]

The USPHS had established detailed regulations for staff conduct on the psychiatric wards to maintain the safety and security of both the employees and the patients. Since psychiatric cases needed constant supervision, the nurses were ordered to "remain constantly on the wards" and were forbidden from leaving at any time "except for meals."[116] For the safety of the hospital staff, ward surgeons were required to inform nurses and attendants of any "suicidal, homicidal, or otherwise dangerous tendencies in the patients."[117] When necessary the staff could initiate a gentle restraint policy, which involved the use of a camisole and a restraining sheet.[118] They could also house patients who were "markedly disturbed" in smaller isolation rooms with the one-on-one supervision of "special attendants."[119]

Knowing how quickly a situation could escalate, Margaret and the USPHS officers had no tolerance for anyone disobeying official regulations. Any staff members, including nurses, who intentionally disregarded the policy was terminated. This policy was initially enacted on October 27, 1915, when Nurse Anna M. Brady was found "guilty of violation of the rules of the station" and relieved of duty.[120]

On October 15, 1915, Anna had reported for day shift duty on the female psychiatric ward, where she had been regularly assigned for weeks. That morning, Anna left the ward and headed to the kitchen, allowing one of her patients to accompany her on the trip. Both actions were clear violations of the posted hospital regulations; however, USPHS officials found her blatant disregard for the safety of that patient and those she left behind on the ward even more egregious. Despite being fully aware that her patient had recently attempted suicide by "jumping in to the ferry boat slip," Anna entered the kitchen alone, leaving her patient unsupervised in an outside corridor.[121] Making matters worse, Anna had also left the ward patients alone and unsupervised. Entering the ward in Anna's absence, USPHS assistant surgeon Howard A. Knox discovered multiple windows open and "the temperature of the room too low for comfort."[122] He also found one patient in an isolation room "stark naked" and "exposed to the elements" while she repeatedly beat her head and hands against the floor.[123]

Upon returning to the ward, Anna was unable to explain her actions and was suspended while a full investigation could be completed. Charges against Anna were clear: she had violated the USPHS regulations regarding proper performance of duties and disobeyed general orders for all employees of the Ellis Island hospitals. USPHS acting assistant surgeon E. K. Sprague ruled that she was "unfitted for the Service" and told Anna that "her usefulness as a nurse in this hospital had terminated."[124] Despite several appeals from the government officials who knew Anna, Surgeon General Rupert Blue supported the decision. Noting Anna's case had been given "careful consideration," Dr. Blue described the nurses' "great responsibility" to prevent harm to psychiatric patients, emphasizing the need for strict attention to medical orders and close supervision to prevent "accidents to these helpless persons."[125]

PSYCHIATRIC TREATMENT FOR SERVICE MEMBERS
After World War I, psychiatrists expanded their understanding of mental illness and their approach to its treatment. Frontline combat in Europe had been traumatic, leaving scores of soldiers battered and broken both physically and

mentally. Following their service, military veterans suffered from a broad range of mental injuries, including direct head trauma, headaches, functional paralysis, hearing loss, depression, insomnia, and memory issues. The term "shell shock" emerged as a catch-all diagnosis for mental injuries sustained during the war, and the high prevalence of war-related psychiatric issues propelled a more active treatment approach among the medical community.

In 1919 Congress charged the USPHS to provide hospital and medical care for all military service members. USPHS surgeon Thomas W. Salmon, who also acted as the medical director of the National Committee of Mental Hygiene, noted an "extraordinary incidence of mental and functional nervous diseases" in combat veterans when he visited Great Britain in 1917.[126] The need for psychiatric services among US veterans would drive "the creation of a rather large neuropsychiatric service" on Ellis Island as Marine Hospital No. 43 admitted greater numbers of military beneficiaries for the care and treatment of mental disorders.[127]

A number of changes were made to Ellis Island hospitals to accommodate these additional psychiatric patients. A building on Island 3 was reassigned for mental illness, increasing bed capacity to a total of forty-six beds. The twenty beds on the closed wards in the "Psychopathic Pavilion" were utilized for "the most disturbed" patients, whereas the "quiet, cooperative patients" were admitted to the open wards of the Contagious Disease Hospital.[128] A consultation service was established with Dr. S. B. Wortis, assistant professor of neurology at New York University, who held a weekly clinic on Ellis Island where each active psychiatric case was presented and discussed.[129] In addition, a referral service was developed under the direction of Dr. Foster Kennedy, a neurosurgeon at Bellevue Hospital. Patients in need of neurosurgery were temporarily transferred to Bellevue for surgery and returned to Ellis Island for recovery and convalescence.

As psychiatric treatment procedures evolved, so did the practice of psychiatric nursing. Therapeutic nursing measures were intended to help a mental patient adjust to their disorder to "function in a manner satisfactory to himself and to society."[130] The care on Ellis Island was no exception. Nurses established daily routines on the psychiatric wards, providing meals, outdoor exercise, and activities at specific times to promote positive wellness habits in their patients.[131] The physician often ordered hydrotherapy treatments for the patients, and nurses initiated and supervised these sessions as needed. Although the immersion of a disturbed patient in a tub of warm water was believed to assist with a broad range of nervous and mental diseases, the nurses needed to ensure their patient's safety at all times. The USPHS physicians prescribed the details of the treatment, including the water temperature, pressure, and the duration of the bath, but the nurses were responsible for following those parameters and for monitoring the patient's vital signs and tolerance of the procedure.[132]

Other treatments were also implemented. Some patients received insulin shock treatments, while others underwent hypnosis. In both instances, the nurses were responsible for carefully monitoring the patients, ensuring that they were safe.[133]

TUBERCULOSIS NURSING AT ELLIS ISLAND

In addition to caring for an increased number of contagious disease and psychiatric cases, the Ellis Island nurses also treated a growing number of tuberculosis (TB) patients. One of the deadliest diseases of all time, tuberculosis, caused by *Mycobacterium tuberculosis*, primarily attacks the lungs and causes severe damage and respiratory complications that can lead to death. Although TB has surged at different times throughout history, the disease spread with epidemic ferocity in cities across the United States during the Industrial Revolution, eventually becoming the leading cause of death in New York City in 1900.[134]

At the time, the poor sanitation and crowded living conditions that characterized tenement districts contributed to the spread of TB among newly arrived immigrants and other working-class poor. Robust public health campaigns and the work of visiting tuberculosis nurses helped to reduce somewhat the prevalence and mortality rates of TB in the first few decades of the twentieth century; however, an effective, curative treatment would not exist until the development of specific antibiotics in the 1950s.[135] Until that time, Ellis Island officials focused their efforts on preventing the spread of TB by immigrant populations. To accomplish this goal, federal immigration policy and USPHS procedures were designed to stop the introduction of TB into the United States by the arriving immigrants. To further restrict the spread of TB, officials deported any immigrant diagnosed with this Class A "dangerous contagious disease."[136]

Mirroring their approach to containing trachoma, USPHS physicians took their time to accurately diagnose TB during the immigrant inspection process. They pulled aside any immigrants who displayed the well-marked pulmonary symptoms—a chronic, productive cough, wheezing, or difficulty breathing—and gave them a more thorough secondary examination. However, they could not make an official diagnosis until the Ellis Island laboratory confirmed the presence of the tubercle bacillus in the sputum. Thus, any suspected TB cases among the immigrant arrivals "were sent as a matter of routine" to the Contagious Disease Hospital on Island 3.[137] The isolated setting and specially designed wards of this hospital were ideal for temporary quarantine. Moreover, with separate rooms explicitly designed to prevent cross infection, care from highly trained and experienced graduate nurses, screened porches where patients had access to fresh breezes off the harbor, and plenty of sunlight and outdoor activity space, the Contagious Disease Hospital also happened to be an ideal therapeutic environment for TB patients.

By 1924 an entire building on the northeast side of the Contagious Disease Hospital had been designated exclusively for the care and treatment of TB cases. That building was necessary. After World War I chronic tuberculosis had emerged as a serious problem among veterans; approximately one-third of all military patients received TB care.[138] Now that the USPHS had assumed responsibility for *all* veteran medical care, the demand for tuberculosis treatment often surpassed the capacity of the local New York marine hospitals. In response, the physicians at the Marine Hospitals at Stapleton and on Staten Island transferred their overflow TB patients to Ellis Island.

The new building contained two wards with a total capacity of thirty-five patient beds. Ward 15, located on the first floor, was set up using the small, cubicle-style isolation design and was "occupied mostly by [Marine Hospital] Service patients."[139] Ward 16, intended for TB overflow or immigrant patients who could afford the cost of treatment, encompassed the second floor and had twenty beds arranged in "a large open ward" design.[140] Landscape upgrades on Ellis Island, which had begun in the immediate postwar period, gradually filled the space between Islands 2 and 3 and created a large outdoor recreation area with walkways where TB patients could exercise. The presence of occupational nurses and vocational therapists at Ellis Island, part of a progressive reform package for detained immigrants, aligned with the specialty treatment protocols encouraged at all USPHS tuberculosis hospitals.[141]

Trained graduate nurses were essential to the success of the required treatment protocols. Nursing care for TB patients required advanced knowledge and specialty training for proper implementation.[142] The nurses needed to instruct their patients on the cause of TB, its risk factors, and the proper ways to mitigate the spread of the disease. They also provided supportive therapies to manage the chronic symptoms.[143] Before assigning a new nurse to the TB wards, Chief Nurse Ellen Cartledge ensured that they were proficient in the performance of all of these duties.

Nursing protocols were detailed and unambiguous. Of primary importance was the prevention of disease spread, so the nurses maintained the procedures for wearing and disposing of gowns and gloves required on every ward of the Contagious Disease Hospital. In addition to implementing these standard infection prevention measures, the nurses saw to it that all the rooms occupied by TB patients were scrubbed daily using soap and hot water; that patients with active symptoms were "kept segregated" from those in latent or quiescent stages; and that any patient with a fever over 38 degrees Celsius remained in bed.[144]

The nurses also encouraged their patients to participate in preventing the spread of the infection by providing them with instructions and the necessary supplies to do so. Each patient received an "ample supply of gauze" and a sputum cup "with an automatic closing top . . . partly filled with a strong antiseptic solution" that was to be carried with them at all times.[145] The nurses instructed the patients to use the gauze to cover their mouths and noses when they coughed or sneezed, and to collect any sputum in the covered, disposable cups. The nurses collected the used gauze and cups daily and immediately sent them to the incinerator.[146]

Supportive care for TB patients involved providing them with fresh air, sunlight, good food, and rest. On Ellis Island, nurses allowed TB patients "as much fresh as air" as was "practicable," while they simultaneously adjusted the open windows to prevent drafts.[147] They also allowed afebrile patients to exercise outside—as long as they followed the physician's prescribed regimen. The nurses taught their patients how to perform breathing exercises meant to help maintain their lung function and prevent further damage to their infected tissue. During open-air sessions a few times per day, they instructed their patients to "breathe through the nose, take a full breath, expand the chest and hold breath a short time, then breathe out."[148]

To support patients' weight gain, nurses and dieticians ensured that they received nourishing foods and incorporated the individual patient's needs and preferences into the meal planning. They strongly encouraged the patients to eat the provided generous portions and consume high-fat foods like milk and eggs. After every meal the nurses required their patients to rest in bed for thirty minutes.[149]

Prior to the discovery of streptomycin in 1944, no definitive cure for tuberculosis was available. As a result, very few patients recovered enough to enjoy an active life after their primary infection. Unfortunately, this was the case for Chief Nurse Margaret Daly.

Margaret first noticed the symptoms of TB in July 1935 but attributed her weight loss and subsequent weakness to the chronic epigastric distress she had been experiencing. As she became weaker and began to cough, Margaret underwent a series of diagnostic tests. Sputum and X-ray results confirmed that she was indeed suffering from tuberculosis, and she was sent to Stapleton Marine Hospital for treatment.

During her first six months of treatment, Margaret showed signs of mild clinical improvement, regaining some of the weight she had lost. However, her case was complicated by her advanced age, chronic hypertension, and bilateral

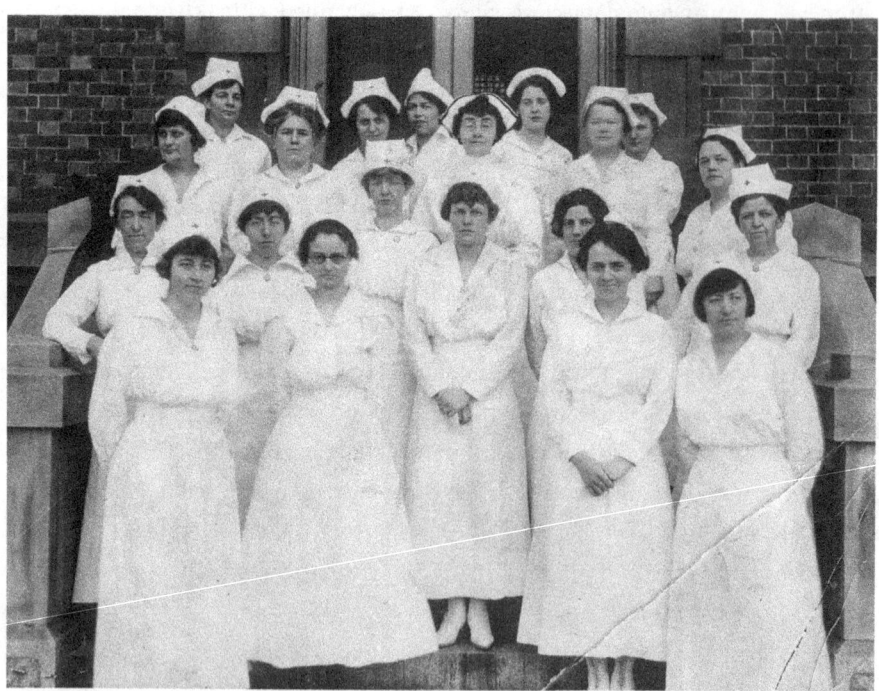

Ellis Island nurses on the steps outside the General Hospital, circa 1930.
Courtesy of the National Park Service, Statue of Liberty National Monument, STLI 24602.

cataracts, and despite her hopes to return to Ellis Island, her physicians declared it was "inadvisable for her to contemplate future work."[150] USPHS acting assistant surgeon C. Fergusen, who oversaw Margaret's care at Stapleton, recommended that she retire in May 1936, only a few months after her initial diagnosis of acute TB in December 1935. Her actual retirement date occurred before May, however. Margaret's tenure on Ellis Island was "discontinued without prejudice" on February 29, 1936, her career officially ending almost thirty-four years after it first began.[151] Just nine months later, on November 5, 1936, Margaret died of complications from tuberculosis.

ANOTHER WARTIME TRANSITION

In the years after Margaret's death, immigration through the Port of New York continued to decline, the rate of hospitalization dropped, and the USPHS further reduced the number of personnel stationed on Ellis Island. Fewer than one thousand patients were treated in Ellis Island hospitals in 1937—a far cry from the peak in 1921, when more than sixteen thousand patients received treatment at Ellis Island.[152]

World events soon brought more changes to the island. When war broke out again in Europe on September 1, 1939, the US Coast Guard was ordered to enforce the terms of the US Neutrality Act by conducting coastal patrols. When the coast guard communicated the need for a strategically located training station to prepare new guardsmen, they eventually selected Ellis Island because it was "ideally situated" to meet current facility needs.[153] By the time the Japanese bombed Pearl Harbor on December 7, 1941, the US Coast Guard training facility was up and running, utilizing a number of buildings across the island. However, the Main Building and hospital complex remained under the jurisdiction of the USPHS. There, physicians and nurses continued their work throughout the war and into the early 1950s.

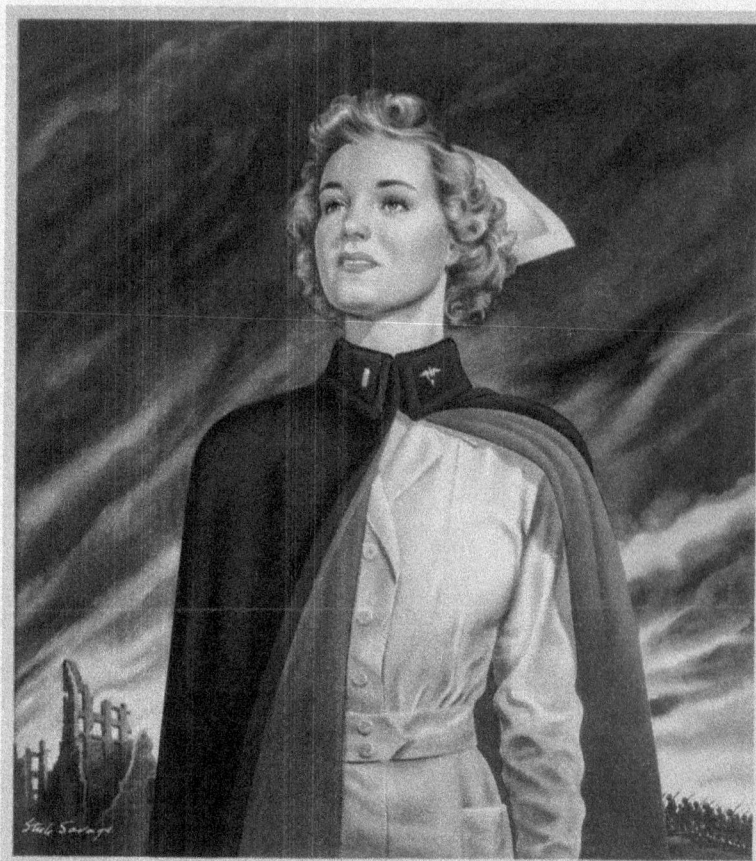

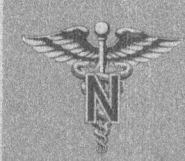

Nurses Are Needed Now!

"Nurses are needed now!" Army Nurse Corps recruitment poster, 1944.
Courtesy of the National Library of Medicine Digital Collections.

CHAPTER 6

WORLD WAR II AND THE END OF A NURSING PRESENCE ON ELLIS ISLAND 1941–1954

REPORT TO ELLIS ISLAND 25 SEPTEMBER 1943. STOP.
BOARD FERRY FROM BATTERY AT 1545 HOURS. STOP[1]

Tearing open the telegram that had just arrived, registered nurse Kathleen Dyer glanced at her orders from the US Public Health Service. Finally! She had been waiting all summer to find out where she would be stationed and when she would go. Settling down on the sofa to read the orders one more time, Kathleen grinned. She had received her first choice of locations! She would be staying on the East Coast rather than heading across the country to Seattle, too far from her ailing mother in Vermont.[2] Kathleen really wanted to be within easy travel distance to her childhood home in case her mother's health deteriorated. Besides, on Ellis Island she'd be just a short ferry ride away from Manhattan. For the twenty-three-year-old who had only been as far as Troy, New York, and Worchester, Massachusetts, where she was now working, the idea of being so close to New York City was exciting. Shopping, theaters, restaurants! Hopefully she'd have some days and evenings free.

Going to the kitchen to get a Coke from the icebox, Kathleen thought of all she had to do to get ready. She only had a few weeks. She still needed a tetanus shot, and she had to buy some new luggage, a raincoat, and three more white uniforms. She had plenty of starched nurses' caps with the black band signifying her RN status, but another pair of Oxford nurses' shoes and a few pairs of hose were certainly called for. She hoped she could find some, given the shortages due to the war. At least she had enough ration coupons. Well, shopping would have to wait. First, she had to let the chief nurse at Memorial Hospital know that she had received orders. After that she'd call her mother.

Kathleen had been, as she put it, "all hyped up" to serve her country ever since the United States had declared war on December 8, 1941, only months after she had graduated from Bishop DeGoesbriand Hospital School of Nursing.[3] Originally, she had planned to join the United States Army Nurse Corps, hoping to serve overseas, but having been convinced that staying in the United States was the better option for her family situation, she had worked domestically for two years. First she had been a private duty nurse in Troy, then worked on a general medical-surgical unit in a hospital in Worchester. This past summer, with two years' nursing experience under her belt, she'd made the decision to enlist in the USPHS instead of the Army Nurse Corps.[4] In a few weeks, Kathleen would report for duty at Marine Hospital No. 43 on Ellis Island.

THE IMPORTANCE OF PLACE IN TIME OF WAR

When the US Coast Guard took over Ellis Island after war broke out in Europe in 1939, coastguardsmen were stationed there as a precautionary measure. However, after the Japanese attacked Pearl Harbor on December 7, 1941, and the United States declared war on Japan and Germany, the Coast Guard's mission changed dramatically. That same day, "all large communities in the area, including New York City, Newark, New Jersey, Bayonne, and Paterson, went on immediate war footing."[5] Ellis Island was no exception. Servicemen now guarded the harbor at the heart of the war effort.

Since then, ominous clouds of war hung over the Upper Bay. The possibility of a German attack on New York Harbor was a real threat—one that stoked tension and fear among the personnel of Ellis Island. As Arthur Dicksen, a coastguardsman who had been stationed on the island since September 1941, noted, "After December 7, the whole atmosphere on the Island changed. . . . More guard duties, more purpose."[6]

The guard duties to which Arthur referred were the result of Ellis Island becoming a temporary detention center for the enemies of the United States. Within hours of the US declaration of war on Japan, special agents of the Federal Bureau of Investigation (FBI) rounded up over one hundred Japanese nationals from New York City and interned them in the main Ellis Island Immigration

Building.[7] Every month since then, FBI agents had brought several hundred enemy aliens to the island. Beginning in the opening months of 1942, the majority of the detainees were of German descent.[8] By 1943 when Kathleen reported for duty on Ellis Island, the daily total of detainees—including German, Japanese, and Italian men and women—hovered around eight hundred.

Most detainees stayed for a few days or weeks before being transported to camps further inland, but some remained on Ellis Island for months or even years.[9] Living conditions were less than ideal. Crowded conditions in makeshift dormitories in the Old Record Rooms on Island 1 fostered the spread of contagious diseases. Meanwhile, detainees spent the few hours they were allowed outside each week "walking in circles round a dreary exercise yard."[10] Adequate nutrition was also a problem as some prisoners refused to eat the strange "American food." Not surprisingly, some of the detainees became sick and required hospital care. And as the numbers of sick increased, so did the need for nurses.

Unfortunately, the increasing demand for nurses on Ellis Island came at the same time that thousands of nurses were needed in military camps at home and abroad. Added to that, most young nurses who wanted to serve their country chose to enlist in the US Army or Navy Nurse Corps rather than in the US Public Health Service. Apparently, the possibility of an assignment overseas was more exciting than being stationed at a marine hospital in the States.

STAFFING FOR WAR

The need for USPHS nurses in other marine hospitals across the United States further decreased the number of nurses available to be assigned to Ellis Island during the first months of the war. Of the nineteen new nurses appointed to the USPHS in January 1942, just two were ordered to Ellis Island. Dorothy Welsh, RN, received her orders first and was soon joined by Lillian Hook.[11] Unfortunately, adding only two nurses to the current staff was not sufficient to meet the hospital's needs. When superintendent of USPHS nurses Kathryn Read inspected Marine Hospital No. 43 in late January 1942, she could clearly see that the hospital needed additional staff.[12] As a result, she ordered Marguerite Jugan, Leona Amon, and Anna Bomberger to report to Ellis Island in March. A few months later, in June 1942, she directed Gertrude Downs to join them.[13]

The arrival of other USPHS nurses on Ellis Island continued into 1943. In January, Anna E. O'Brien reported for duty at Marine Hospital No. 43.[14] Ethyland

Kuhns followed in February, Agnes D. Avent in March, and Catherine Feeney in April.[15] In May 1943 three more nurses, Dorothy Sitcer, Edith Ibbott, and Doris Squires, joined the workforce.[16] Later, other nurses received their orders to report to Ellis Island. Among these were Ina Sausville (Delaney), Lenore Rainey, Virginia Vesh, Irene Bosco, Mary Madden, and finally, in the summer of 1943, Kathleen Dyer.[17]

REPORTING FOR DUTY

Leaving Boston by train on the morning of September 25, 1943, Kathleen Dyer traveled to Penn Station in New York City, then made her way down to the Battery at the southernmost tip of Manhattan Island. She was just in time to catch the 3:45 p.m. ferry to Ellis Island. Taking a deep breath, she gripped the railing as she stumbled up the gangplank, the metal platform bumping against the dock with the rise and fall of the choppy water. She certainly hoped the water would not be this rough every time she made the commute.

Holding onto support poles and railings, Kathleen wobbled to the nearest bench and took a seat. Whew. Exciting as it was, this ferry crossing also filled her with anxiety. Catching sight of the island in the distance as the boat chugged across the river, Kathleen began to appreciate how different life would be working on Ellis Island rather than on the mainland. Marine Hospital No. 43 was certainly isolated. And yet it was situated in a harbor bustling with activity. More than forty shipyards lined the coast. And, in addition to the usual ocean liners, ferries, barges, and tugboats, all types of military vessels crowded the open bay. Troop transport ships, aircraft carriers, battle cruisers, and coast guard cutters were seemingly everywhere.[18] For Kathleen, the gravity of her oath to the United States suddenly took on new meaning. What was she getting herself into?

Within minutes the ferry docked on Ellis Island. Cautiously stepping onto the bouncing metal gangway, Kathleen paused and scanned the wharf. Someone was supposed to be there to meet her. Relieved to see that another young nurse, clad in her white uniform, cap, and navy-blue cape, was waving to get her attention, Kathleen returned the wave with a smile.

Having made brief introductions, the two nurses were ready to move on. The welcoming nurse's job was to lead Kathleen to the chief nurse's office, show her to her sleeping quarters, and give her a tour of the hospital.[19] Hopefully, she would also reassure Kathleen that she had made a good decision when she enlisted in the US Public Health Service.

The first order of business was registration. Crossing the bridge to Islands 2 and 3 (by this time connected by landfill), the nurses made their way to the Contagious Disease Hospital where Kathleen had been told to check in. Entering the chief nurse's office, Kathleen noted the gleaming wood floors, large windows, and fourteen-foot-high ceiling framed with mahogany crown molding. The room was impressive, reflecting the chief nurse's position. Just standing in front of the desk proved to be a bit intimidating, and Kathleen had to remind herself to take some deep breaths. She was really doing this!

A half hour later, after completing a plethora of government forms and receiving the keys to her room, Kathleen and her escort headed down a long corridor to the nurses' quarters at the back of Island 3. Settling in to her new accommodations was Kathleen's next order of business.[20]

Entering the small building that served as the nurses' dormitory, the two nurses soon found Kathleen's room, located in one of the four-bedroom suites on

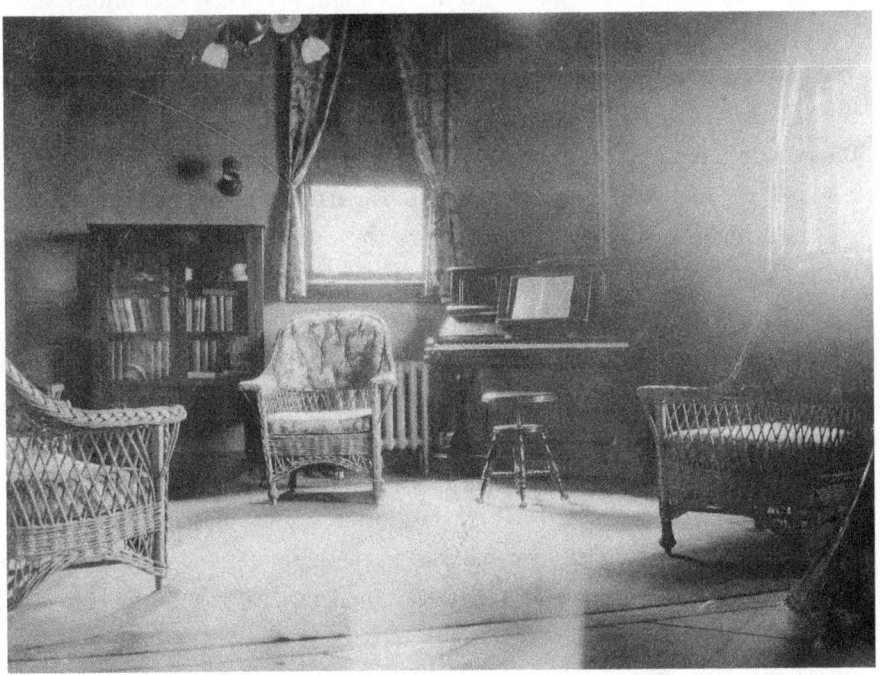

View of the common room in the nurses' dormitory on Ellis Island.
Courtesy of the National Park Service, Statue of Liberty National Monument, STLI 5052.

the second floor. In each suite, two single bedrooms were connected by a shared bathroom—complete with a cast-iron tub. A shared living room with a mahogany-trimmed ceiling made up the center portion. Throughout the suite, large windows afforded light and ventilation. Still clutching her suitcase, Kathleen stopped to take a glimpse out the window. She could see the shore of New Jersey just across the Hudson River.[21] It wasn't exactly the best view, but at least she could see some boats making their way down the river. At any rate, the breeze coming through the screen was delightful!

Turning away from the window, Kathleen dropped her luggage on the bed. She would unpack later. Meeting some of the other nurses assigned to Marine Hospital No. 43 and getting something to eat were the next items on her agenda. Heading back down the stairs, the two nurses exited the building to walk to the dining hall. It was almost time for dinner.

Minutes later, Ina M. Sausville, a 1934 graduate of St. Vincent's Hospital in Worchester, Massachusetts, crossed the lawn to join them. Having made introductions all around, Kathleen soon discovered that Ina had been stationed in Baltimore with the USPHS but, hating the city's summer heat and humidity, she had applied for a transfer to "any location in the northeast."[22] Once that transfer was granted, Ina had moved to New York in 1942. At first, Ina had stayed in the nurses' quarters on Ellis Island. However, as additional nurses arrived to staff the hospital and space in the nurses' quarters proved inadequate to meet the demand, Ina had volunteered to move to an apartment on Staten Island. Like other staff members who chose to lodge in nearby communities, she commuted to the island by ferry.

Making their way into the nurses' dining room, Kathleen and her new friends stopped to check the dinner menu posted on the wall. They had a choice: pot roast with noodles or lamb stew with potatoes.[23] Well, that was easy. Having been a New Englander all her life, Kathleen chose the pot roast. At least tonight the food would be familiar; everything else was strange and new.

Ah, it looked like tomorrow's breakfast menu was also posted. The choices were oatmeal or scrambled eggs with bacon—both entrées served with toast, juice, and coffee. Planning ahead, Kathleen thought she'd choose the eggs—as long as they weren't the powdered ones typically allowed with government-issued rationing coupons. In general, she surmised that the meals would be bland but filling; not much variety. Kathleen had been hoping to sample some

New York cuisine, but for the most part that would not occur—at least not on the island. The exception: sometimes there would be "a little area [on the island] where you could get a hot dog."[24]

Picking up her fork to sample the pot roast, Kathleen listened to the other nurses explain the benefits of living on the island, a world unto itself. Not only did the nurses eat, sleep, and work on the tiny island—they also spent most of their free time there. Movies and dances were held onsite in the recreation building only steps from the hospital. Tennis courts were also available for the nurses' use. Even the nurses' laundry was done on the island. Their white uniforms, pajamas, and undergarments—all labeled with their names—were washed and dried in the hospital's laundry facilities before being returned to their rightful owners.

"ROUTINE" NURSING WORK

After a restless night in unfamiliar surroundings, Kathleen reported to the senior ward nurse on Ward 20, one of the wards for patients with either medical or surgical problems. Listening to the morning report, she realized that she was well prepared for her new assignment. In fact, the work here would be less demanding than it had been at Worchester Memorial Hospital: Marine Hospital No. 43 only admitted patients who had non–life-threatening injuries or medical conditions.[25] Anyone who was critically ill or needed surgery was sent to Stapleton Marine Hospital on Staten Island.[26] According to the information provided by the night nurse, most of the patients in Marine Hospital No. 43 had "orthopedic problems, colds, minor injuries, and chest problems." Indeed, the work would be "quite routine," just as Ina Sausville had told her the night before.[27] According to Ina, with the exception of one patient with acute abdominal pain whom she had transferred to Stapleton, the care she had given on Ellis Island over the past year was "more or less custodial"—there were "no big things."[28]

As Ina reported, men with orthopedic problems took up most of the nurses' time.[29] Using the skills they had developed in their training programs, the nurses inspected fingers and toes "recently encased in plaster" casts and reported any pain, abnormal odors, or symptoms of coldness, pallor, blueness, edema, and numbness. They lifted their patients carefully and turned them frequently to relieve any pressure points on their skin. In summer, when heat and humidity pervaded the island, the nurses used fans to keep the patients cool in their plaster casts.[30] After a cast was removed, the nurses gently washed the area to remove the "yellow exudate that was partly dead skin" and applied cocoa butter to promote healing.[31]

Discussing her work on any given eight-hour shift, Kathleen later described the typical schedule: "First thing, we would count the drugs [narcotics], and then make rounds to see the fifteen or sixteen patients on the ward, giving medications and 'syringe injections.'"[32] The many injections Kathleen administered included penicillin. Early in the war, the new antibiotic had been released to the military and was used to treat a wide variety of infections. Most often the new "wonder drug" was used for infected wounds or pneumonia. It was also the drug of choice for the treatment of syphilis and gonorrhea.[33]

As was the case in other US hospitals in the 1940s, Kathleen's work included taking patients' temperatures, monitoring their pulse rate and respirations, and checking their blood pressures. Since the late nineteenth century, nurses had been making close observations of their patients' conditions, using their own eyes as well as devices such as the thermometer. By the 1940s, they were also using blood pressure cuffs—devices that until the mid-1930s had been used only by physicians. Now, standard nursing practice included checking the patients' temperatures and blood pressures, charting them accurately, and reporting any problems to the physician.[34]

SOLUTIONS TO THE NURSING SHORTAGE

Given the shortage of nurses during the war, Kathleen and her colleagues relied on hospital attendants to help them complete the myriad tasks they had to accomplish each day. Among the attendants was Isaac Cox, one of the first Black male hospital attendants on the island. Reflecting on his work in the Ellis Island hospital in the early 1940s, Cox recalled, "I reported to the head nurse each day, then did my assigned chores—washing patients, [making] beds, and helping the nurses with whatever needed to be done."[35] Cox was career conscious; during the war he certified as a Licensed Practical Nurse (LPN) under a program for "waiver nurses."[36] Like hospital attendants, LPNs were essential providers of nursing care during World War II.

As the war dragged on, the nursing shortage in the United States reached a critical level. By August 1944 the military was calling for one thousand nurses a month for the army and five hundred for the navy, further depleting the

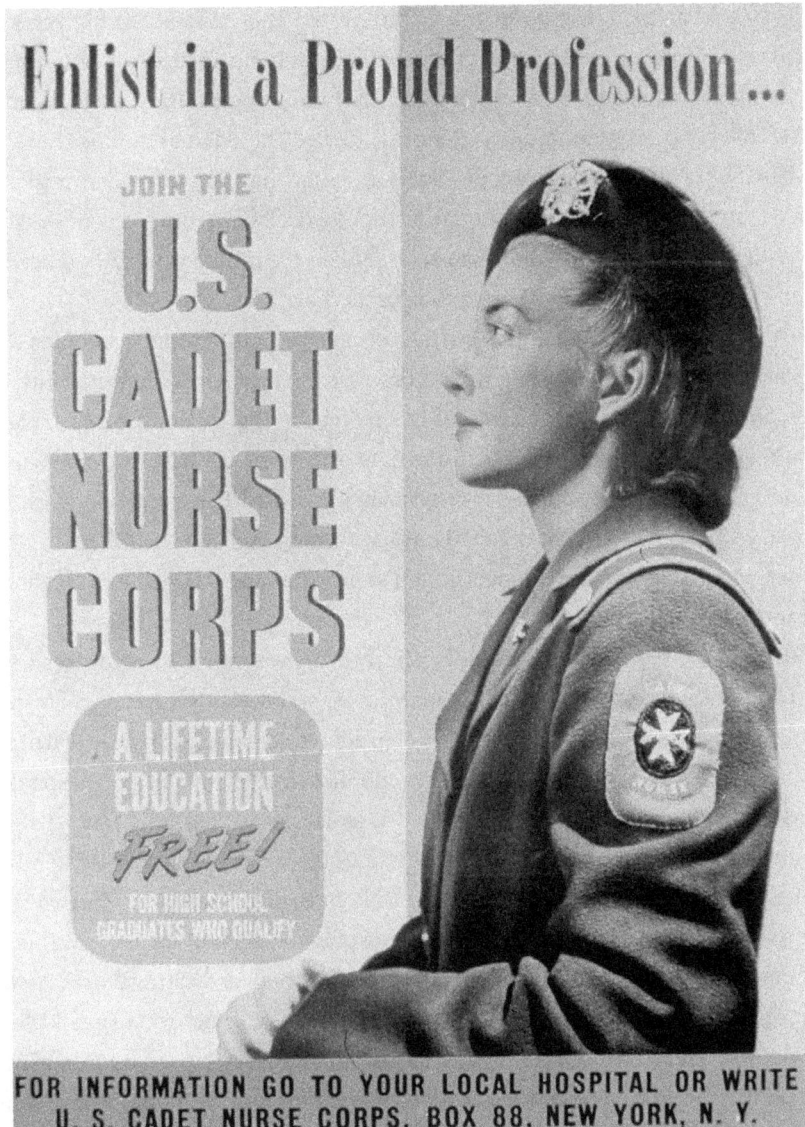

"Enlist in a proud profession . . ." U.S. Cadet Nurse Corps recruitment poster, 1943.
Courtesy of the National Library of Medicine Digital Collections.

number of nurses available to work in civilian and marine hospitals. The hospital on Ellis Island was no exception. To meet its staffing needs, the administration of Marine Hospital No. 43 recruited senior students from the United States Cadet Nurse Corps.

As early as 1942, the government recognized that nurse training schools across the country would have to graduate more students to meet the increasing demands for nurses in both military and civilian hospitals. In order to accomplish this goal, on June 15, 1943, Congress passed the Bolton Act, creating the United States Cadet Nurse Corps. The legislation not only provided nursing schools with funds for instructional facilities and faculty but also subsidized the education of students who promised to serve in a military or civilian health agency after graduation for the duration of the war.

A recruitment campaign followed. To convince young women to enter the profession of nursing, the government promised to provide cadets with tuition, fees, and books along with a monthly stipend during their training. Cadets would also receive a smart dress uniform of gray wool, complete with a stylish "Montgomery" beret and a cadet insignia arm patch.[37] The campaign worked. On May 14, 1944, over ninety-five thousand women pledged themselves to the Cadet Nurse Corp and the US government to provide "essential nursing services" for the duration of the war.[38]

One of the requirements for cadets in training was to fill in for nurses who had gone to war. During the last six months of their senior year of nurse training, cadets took on the responsibilities of graduate nurses—essentially learning on the job. Some cadets spent these six months in their hometown hospitals, working as charge nurses on the wards or as assistants in operating and delivery rooms. However, since the US Cadet Nurse Corps encouraged schools to offer cadets affiliations beyond what was available in their hometowns, some cadets completed their senior year outside of the hospital in which they were training.[39] Of these, some worked in psychiatric hospitals, others at Visiting Nurse Associations, military camps, tuberculosis sanatoria, or large urban hospitals. Still others worked for the USPHS on American Indian reservations and in marine hospitals.[40] At least one—Irene Sabo, a young woman from Ohio—was sent to Ellis Island.[41]

IRENE SABO, CADET NURSE

Checking her mail for the tenth time in the last two days, Irene Sabo finally saw the letter she had been waiting for. The return address was the Massillon State Hospital School of Nursing. Ripping open the envelope and removing the official letter, she scanned the first sentence: "It is with pleasure that I write to inform you of your admission to the Cadet program at the Massillon State Hospital School of Nursing, beginning September 6, 1943."[42] Hurray! She would notify her employer of her plans to resign from the Hoover Vacuum Cleaner Factory when she reported for her shift in the morning. She was going to be a cadet nurse!

Sitting at the table, Irene read through the rest of the letter's instructions. She would be a pre-cadet for the first nine months of the program—now, because of the war, shortened to two and a half years instead of the usual three. Then, she would be a junior cadet for the remainder of the abbreviated curriculum.[43] During her senior year, she would be assigned to a civilian or military hospital that needed nurses. During training, Irene would be required to wear the cadet dress uniform only for special events. For the most part, she would wear her regular student uniform. Best of all, the government would pay for all her school expenses. All she had to do was pledge to serve her country "for the duration of the war" or for a year after graduation. Irene was eager to get started.

The two years training in Ohio sped by. During that time, in addition to theoretical nursing knowledge, Irene learned to assist in the operating room, give bed baths and backrubs, and monitor patients for any change in their condition. She also learned how to skillfully complete "over 200 nursing procedures" and how to properly administer medications.[44] She was ready for her senior affiliation.

Assigned to Marine Hospital No. 43 in the spring of 1945, Irene soon found herself packing for the trip to New York. A week later she took the ferry to Ellis Island, registered with the chief nurse, settled into her room, and reported for duty.

As a senior student, Irene had the knowledge and skills she needed to care for hospitalized patients. Relying on what she had learned in her time at Massillon State Hospital, Irene adapted easily to the work. For the most part, she was already familiar with the treatments and medications in use at the marine hospital. What she had not expected, however, was that she would be asked to assist with the administration of electric shock treatments in the psychiatric ward when doctors needed an extra pair of hands. Irene had actually never seen the procedure. Up until this time, hydrotherapy and insulin shock had been used to treat psychiatric patients. In 1945 however, electric shock therapy was the treatment of choice for schizophrenia and depression.[45]

Irene's time as a senior cadet was not all work. Like other cadets stationed in New York City, she took some time to visit museums, attend theaters, and shop in department stores in Manhattan. She also watched movies and went to dances in the recreation hall.

Meeting coastguardsmen, USPHS physicians, and dentists stationed on the island was one of the perks for the young cadet. As a fellow cadet nurse assigned to a hospital in Manhattan put it, "We appreciated the abundance of dates" given the availability of so many service men in the city.[46] In Irene's case, she didn't even need to venture off the island; she met her future husband in the staff cafeteria. Dr. Burton Kane was a dental intern in the US Public Health Service.[47]

THE POSTWAR YEARS

After World War II ended in June 1945, changes in government policies once again influenced the nurses' role on Ellis Island. Enemy aliens were freed, and for almost a year Marine Hospital No. 43 nurses cared only for US coastguardsmen and returning soldiers. The nature of their patients changed once again, however, when the government decommissioned the Ellis Island Coast Guard Training Station in 1946. For the next few years, the Ellis Island nurses cared not only for US troops, merchant marines, and injured coastguardsmen but also for any steerage-class immigrants who arrived in New York Harbor by ship.[48] During that time, the number of patients admitted to the hospital each year averaged about forty-five hundred.[49]

As air travel became more common and more Europeans sought entry into the United States via airports rather than in the Port of New York, the cost of maintaining an immigration station and immigrant hospitals on Ellis Island became prohibitive. Given this reality, in 1947 US immigration commissioner Ugo Carusi recommended to Congress that the government abandon Ellis Island and transfer its activities to the Immigration Service Building in New York City. In his testimony before the Committee on Appropriations, the commissioner argued that closing Ellis Island would save the government up to $300,000 a year. He also noted that during recent months "his service had been concentrating their efforts against illegal entry of foreigners along the Mexican border." According to Carusi, the situation at the border was "causing much difficulty" for local authorities.[50] Despite Carusi's recommendations, however, four years passed before Congress closed the Ellis Island hospitals.

In the meantime, USPHS nurses staffed both the Ellis Island General Hospital on Island 2 and the Contagious Disease Hospital on Island 3, treating three hundred to four hundred patients each month. By 1949, in addition to the small psychiatric ward on Island 2, Wards 13, 14, 17, 18, and 23 of the Contagious Disease Hospital had been repurposed and classified as "mental wards," with Ward 13 being set aside for violent and acutely disturbed patients and Ward 23 designated for "mental-TB" patients.[51] As Dr. James Baker, director of neuropsychiatric services from 1949–1951, described it, "We had six wards containing a total of 200 beds for acute psychiatric patients on Island #3—the only psych services around for Coast Guard and merchant marines."[52] In these wards Baker and his colleagues continued to treat psychiatric patients with electric shock therapy.

The administration of electric shock treatments required at least six staff: a physician, a nurse, and four assistants. Thus, like Irene Sabo had done earlier in the decade, nurses working on the psychiatric wards assisted with these complicated therapies, preparing patients before the treatments were given and monitoring them closely during the shock treatments and after the procedures. It was not an easy task. Later Dr. Baker remarked on the benefits of the nurses' help, noting, "We were fortunate in having nurses that were trained to deal with psychiatric patients."[53]

Meanwhile, in the other wards of the Contagious Disease Hospital, a different cadre of USPHS nurses cared for patients with tuberculosis. The contagious respiratory disease was quite prevalent at the time. From October 1948 to 1951, five to eight immigrants per month were "detained on medical hold" for suspected tuberculosis.[54] Treating these patients was a challenge. As they had been doing since the turn of the twentieth century, nurses saw to it that TB patients received adequate nourishment, that they rested every day, and that they spent hours outdoors on the covered porches, taking in as much fresh air as possible. Following physicians' orders, the nurses routinely gave these patients streptomycin and para-aminosalicylic acid, the two drugs recognized in 1945 as cutting-edge therapies for the devastating disease.[55]

ELLIS ISLAND CLOSES

The nurses' time on the island after the war was short-lived. "In the interest of economy and efficiency," after New Year's Day, January 1951, no new patients were admitted to the Ellis Island hospitals.[56] A few months later, on March 1, 1951, the Ellis Island hospitals closed their doors for the final time.[57] For the next three years, only a few nurses remained to staff the island's small dispensary. Patients requiring hospitalization were sent to the mainland. In 1954 the government evacuated Ellis Island, leaving the immigration station, the hospitals, and other buildings abandoned, the nurses and others working for the USPHS all but forgotten.

CONCLUSION

When the Ellis Island hospitals closed and the nurses left, little evidence of their physical presence on the island remained. Any documentation of their activities also vanished as the island fell into disuse and disrepair and the story of the "hospital for immigrants" fell from collective memory. What nurses did leave behind, however, was a legacy of care for hundreds of thousands of immigrants, thousands of merchant seamen, coastguardsmen, military veterans, and the "enemy aliens" detained on the island during the First and Second World Wars.

That care was shaped by the hospital's geographic location on a tiny man-made island in New York Harbor—a world unto itself but one that changed with a shifting social and political environment during two world wars and with seemingly constant alterations to the federal immigration policy. That legacy of care was also shaped by the nurses' place in the military and medical hierarchy of the United States Public Health Service. Working on Ellis Island, nurses had to balance the demands of two competing pledges: their allegiance to their patients as caring professionals and their oath to the US government.

From 1892 to the shutting of the hospital doors in 1951, the Ellis Island nurses worked in one of the largest USPHS hospitals in the United States. Using state-of-the-art scientific knowledge and medical equipment, these professional nurses collaborated with physicians, social workers, dieticians, ward maids, pharmacists, lab technicians, and others to care for over 1.2 million patients.[1] For the most part nurses were invisible caregivers, but they were also indispensable. Without them, the USPHS physicians could not have provided the care they did. Over the years, nurses assisted in surgeries and obstetrical deliveries, cared for newborn infants and their mothers, used their knowledge and skills to attend both adults and children with contagious diseases, and assisted in the long-term treatment of military service members. They managed and manipulated the therapeutic environment to enhance the supportive treatments that had been ordered by physicians, and expertly administered drugs, fresh air therapy, and special diets to all of their patients.

During the height of immigration from 1902 to 1914, the nurses balanced their ethical duty to care with their obligations to protect the health of the nation. Following directives from the commissioner of immigration, they treated immigrants with respect and kindness, sometimes providing children with small treats and gentle caresses. Their duty to care also meant following physicians' orders, and nurses frequently administered painful treatments to treat diseases like favus and trachoma. Occasionally they assisted in the enforcement of immigration laws, which ran counter to their patients' hope to enter the United States.

Working in the Contagious Disease Hospital after it opened in 1911, the nurses isolated patients to prevent the spread of illnesses like measles, scarlet fever, whooping cough, chicken pox, and diphtheria. Adhering to strict protocols, the nurses navigated the spaces within their profession and within the public health hierarchy, reporting to nursing supervisors and USPHS physicians alike.[2] For the most part, the Ellis Island nurses worked on wards without direct physician supervision, afforded the professional respect and independence that came with graduate nursing. Armed only with supportive therapies and keen skills in observation, these nurses cared for critically ill patients, using their knowledge and clinical judgment to determine when to escalate care.

World War I provided a brief interlude in nursing activities on Ellis Island. The island was the ideal location from which nurses could deploy to Europe, and for nine months, from June 1917 until March 1918, Island 3 was used as a mobilization site for nurses. At the same time, Chief Nurse Margaret Daly remained on Island 2, supervising the care of a few immigrants, as well as captured German prisoners, merchant marines, and injured soldiers returning from Europe. When the army requisitioned the hospitals in the spring of 1918, the nurses' role was affected once more as Margaret Daly and the majority of the Ellis Island nurses transferred to the Marine Hospital at Stapleton, New York, and the army nurses were forced to mobilize from the mainland. Finally, in June 1919 when the army evacuated Ellis Island after World War I, Margaret returned as chief nurse to the Ellis Island General Hospital, only to face the fourth wave of the deadly influenza pandemic that had circled the world in 1918.

In the decades of the 1920s and '30s, nurses working for the USPHS on Ellis Island were once again tasked with protecting the health of the nation, shifting their activities to conform to more restrictive immigration laws. They assisted with surgeries, helped with obstetrical deliveries, and continued to care for patients with contagious illness. These decades also changed the patient mix on Ellis Island. Since the restrictive new quota laws drastically reduced the number of immigrant patients, the government tasked the USPHS and the Marine Hospital system to provide all specialty care to military servicemen. Ellis Island nurses, now officially working at Marine Hospital No. 43, began to treat military men and their families for psychiatric disorders and chronic illnesses like tuberculosis. The nursing staff also lost their longtime leader, Margaret Daly, to complications from tuberculosis in 1936.

Finally, from 1940 to 1951 the Ellis Island nurses provided care for coast-guardsmen and their families, enemy aliens interned on the island, and the few immigrants who continued to arrive by ship. The nurses did so with courage, compassion, and allegiance to the United States, adhering to immigration laws whether or not they agreed with them, all while serving patients without regard to race, gender, age, and ethnicity. In her memoir, written just before her death in 1936, Margaret Daly best summed up the Ellis Island nursing experience by saying:

> My life has been greatly enriched through contact with Ellis Island—
> meeting and assisting all sorts and conditions of men, women and
> children from the very ends of the earth. The Island is small but what a
> host of people have tarried here and have received encouragement and
> help. I have known so many of them and their joys and their sorrows were
> mine. Many have come back again and again to visit the hospital and to
> express their thanks for the attention extended to them by doctors and
> nurses. Gratitude thus acknowledged is perhaps the most precious of all.[3]

The story of these nurses—using their names and their own words—provides a more complete picture of the history of Ellis Island than has been previously drawn. Their story also makes visible the essential role they played not only in caring for the newcomers but also in protecting the health of the

American public. The nurses' story also provides valuable information for the United States today as the government seeks to address the needs of thousands of immigrants arriving at its borders. The lesson is clear: Homeland Security officials should not overlook the role that nurses can play in those efforts; nurses are indispensable in the provision of safe, effective, and compassionate care.

NOTES

INTRODUCTION

1. Emma Lazarus, "The New Colossus," 1883, Library of Congress, https://www.loc.gov/exhibits/haventohome/images/hh0041s.jpg.

2. Susan Reverby, *Ordered to Care: The Dilemma of American Nursing, 1850–1945* (Cambridge: Cambridge University Press, 1987).

3. Narrative nonfiction, also referred to as literary nonfiction or creative nonfiction, refers to all writing that is based on facts that has been composed with specific attention to the craft of writing, employing literary techniques to describe people and events that actually occurred. See Howard Markel, "'The Eyes Have It': Trachoma, the Perception of Disease, the United States Public Health Service, and the American Jewish Immigration Experience, 1897–1924," *Bulletin of the History of Medicine* 74, no. 3 (Fall 2000): 525–60. Markel recreates the USPHS inspection and hospital treatment experience of Rabbi Chaim Goldenbaum, an eastern European immigrant who was processed through the Ellis Island Station in 1916. See also Laurel Thatcher Ulrich, *A Midwife's Tale: The Life of Martha Ballard, Based on Her Diary, 1785–1812* (New York: Vintage, 2010) and Lindsey Fitzharris, *The Butchering Art: Joseph Lister's Quest to Transform the Grisly World of Victorian Medicine* (New York: Scientific American, 2017).

CHAPTER 1

1. "Landed on Ellis Island," *New York Times*, January 2, 1892, http://timesmachine.nytimes.com/timesmachine/1892/01/01/issue.html.

2. In 1892 newspaper articles did not name individual authors; therefore, the name of the journalist remains unknown. It was not common practice to give authors a byline until 1925.

3. "Landed on Ellis," 2.

4. "Landed on Ellis," 2.

5. Howard Markel, "'Knocking out Cholera': Cholera, Class, and Quarantine in New York City, 1892," *Bulletin of the History of Medicine* 69, no. 3 (Fall 1995): 420–57 (quote p. 439). See also Howard Markel, *Quarantine: East European Jewish Immigrants and the New York City Epidemics of 1892* (Baltimore: Johns Hopkins University Press, 1997), 7. Nurses had been working in the quarantine hospitals for quite some time.

According to Markel, in 1892 ten nurses worked in the quarantine hospital on Swinburne Island.

6. "Landed on Ellis," 2.

7. "Landed on Ellis," 2.

8. "Landed on Ellis," 2.

9. "Landed on Ellis," 2.

10. "First Foot on Ellis Island," *New York Sun*, January 2, 1892; see also "The First Emigrant," *Pittsburg Dispatch*, January 2, 1892.

11. Julian Ralph, "Landing the Immigrants," *Harper's Weekly*, October 24, 1891, 821.

12. US Congress, *An Act in Amendment to the Various Acts Relative to Immigration and the Importation of Aliens under Contract or Agreement to Perform Labor* (1891 Immigration Act), 51st Congress, Session 2, chapter 551, 26 Statutes-at-Large 1084, March 3, 1891. The United States Marine Hospital Service was renamed the United States Public Health and Marine Hospital Service in 1902, and again in 1912 as the United States Public Health Service. The standard history of the USPHS remains Ralph Chester Williams, *The United States Public Health Service: 1798–1950* (Bethesda, MD: Commissioned Officers Association of the United States Public Health Service, 1951). See also Elizabeth Yew, "Medical Inspection of Immigrants at Ellis Island, 1891–1924," *Bulletin of New York Academy of Medicine* 56, no. 5 (1980): 488–89.

13. Edward Oxford, "Hope, Tears, and Remembrance," *American History Illustrated*, September/October 1990, 28–49 (quote pp. 38–39).

14. Frank L. White, "Barriers against Invisible Foes," *Frank Leslie's Popular Monthly* 33 (January–June 1892): 662–72.

15. Ralph, "Landing the Immigrants," 821.

16. Ralph, "Landing the Immigrants," 821.

17. Ralph, "Landing the Immigrants," 821.

18. US Congress, 1891 Immigration Act. Immigrants were also interviewed by an immigration inspector (a nonmedical officer) who tried to identify any other mandatory excludable cases: convicts, polygamists, or any person who needed assistance from others.

19. William Williams, "Ellis Island: Its Organization and Some of Its Work," as cited in Harlan D. Unrau, *Historic Resource Study, Ellis Island, Statue of Liberty National Monument New York–New Jersey*, vol. 2 (Denver: US Department of the Interior National Park Service, 1984), 491. Using information they had obtained from the medical certificate and the answers to interview questions, the Board of Special Inquiry ultimately determined whether to admit or deport the detained immigrant.

20. "Gateway of the Continent," *Brooklyn Daily Eagle*, January 5, 1896.

21. "Caring for Immigrants," *New York Times*, June 16, 1897, https://www.archive.nytimes.com.

22. Susan Reverby, *Ordered to Care: The Dilemma of American Nursing, 1850–1945* (Cambridge: Cambridge University Press, 1987).

23. Michelle Hehman, "The Rise of a Profession: 'An Art and a Science,'" in *History of Professional Nursing in the United States*, ed. Arlene Keeling, Michelle Hehman, and

John Kirchgessner (New York: Springer Publishing, 2018), 44–72 (early sketches of the hospital facilities on Hoffman and Swineburn Islands also include female nurses in their professional uniforms, further supporting this claim); "A Nursing School," *Friends of the Ruin*, accessed April 18, 2022, https://www.theruin.org /history-nursing.

24. For more on this topic see Reverby, *Ordered to Care*, 86–87.

25. Darlene Clark Hine, *Black Women in White: Racial Conflict and Cooperation in the Nursing Profession, 1890–195* (Indianapolis: Indiana University Press, 1989), 9.

26. Reverby, *Ordered to Care*.

27. Patricia D'Antonio, *American Nursing: A History of Knowledge, Authority, and the Meaning of Work* (Baltimore: Johns Hopkins University Press, 2010), 28–53.

28. Office of the supervising surgeon general, Marine Hospital Service, "Facts Showing the Quasi-Military Character of the U.S. Marine Hospital Service," August 7, 1896, 1; Bob Hope Memorial Library, Archives and Special Collections, National Park Service at Ellis Island.

29. Markel, *Quarantine*, 23.

30. Office of the supervising surgeon general, "Facts Showing the Quasi-military Character," 1.

31. Hehman, "Rise of a Profession," 44–72. See also Reverby, *Ordered to Care*.

32. J. Tracy Stakely, *Cultural Landscape Report for Ellis Island* (Brookline, MA: National Park Service, Olmsted Center for Landscape Preservation, May 2003), 27–29.

33. Florence Nightingale, *Notes on Hospitals* (London: John W. Parker and Son, 1859), 8.

34. D. J. Milton Miller, MD, "The Hygiene of the Sick Room," *Trained Nurse and Hospital Review* 14 (1895): 135–39 (quote p. 136). See also Stakely, *Cultural Landscape Report*, 27–29.

35. *Encyclopedia Britannica*, s.v. "Robert Koch, German Bacteriologist," accessed April 5, 2022, https://www.britannica.com/biography/Robert-Koch.

36. David Rosner, *Hives of Sickness: Public Health and Epidemics in New York City* (New Brunswick, NJ: Rutgers University Press, 1995), 13.

37. Don K. Nakayama, "Antisepsis and Asepsis and How They Shaped Modern Surgery," *American Surgery* 84, no. 6 (June 2018): 766–71.

38. Arlene Keeling, personal observations of equipment during tour of the abandoned hospitals, Ellis Island, March 8, 2017. See also Lori Conway, *Forgotten Ellis Island: The Extraordinary Story of America's Immigrant Hospital* (New York: HarperCollins, 2007).

39. Joel D. Howell, *Technology in the Hospital: Transforming Patient Care in the Early Twentieth Century* (Baltimore: Johns Hopkins University Press, 1995), 52, 273.

40. Margarete Sandelowski, "'Making the Best of Things': Technology in American Nursing, 1870–1940," *Nursing History Review* 5, no. 1 (1997): 3–22 (quote p. 5).

41. Anna Fullerton, "The Training of Nurses," *Trained Nurse and Hospital Review* 16, nos. 3–6 (March 1896): 132–35 (quote p. 132).

42. Sandelowski, "Making the Best of Things," 3–22.

43. Mary V. Clymer, "Professor Ashurst on the Duties of a Nurse at a Surgical Operation, January 8, 1889," *Mary V. Clymer Lecture Notes, 1887–1889*, MC-16, vol. 1, Barbara Bates

Center for the Study of the History of Nursing, University of Pennsylvania School of Nursing (hereafter BBCSHN, UPENN).

44. Kathleen Latta, "The Clinical Thermometer," *Trained Nurse and Hospital Review* 17, no. 11 (November 1896): 585.

45. D'Antonio, *American Nursing*, 44.

46. Mary V. Clymer, "Lecture Delivered by Dr. William Pepper to the Probationers of the Training School on November 11, 1887," *Mary V. Clymer Lecture Notes, 1887–1889*, MC-16, vol. 1, BBCSHN, UPENN.

47. "The Diet Kitchen: Beverages for the Sick," *Trained Nurse and Hospital Review* 14, no. 4 (June 1895): 222.

48. "Diet Kitchen," 222. For "Breakfast cocoa" made by Walter Baker & Company, see *Trained Nurse and Hospital Review* 16, nos. 3–6 (1896): 168.

49. Mary Cadwalader Jones, "The Training of a Nurse," *Scribner's Magazine* 8, no. 5 (1890): 613–25 (quote p. 620).

50. Advertisements, *Trained Nurse and Hospital Review* 15 (1896): n.p.

51. "Diet Kitchen," 222.

52. "Diet Kitchen," 222.

53. Arlene Keeling, *Nursing and the Privilege of Prescription, 1893–2000* (Columbus: Ohio State University Press, 2007), 13. See also *Trained Nurse and Hospital Review* 16 (1896): 168.

54. Jones, "Training of a Nurse," 617.

55. Jones, "Training of a Nurse," 621.

56. Jones, "Training of a Nurse," 620.

57. "This Month on Ellis Island," National Park Service, accessed April 26, 2022, https://www.nps.gov.

58. J. S. Taylor, "Obstetric Nursing in New York Maternity Hospital," *Trained Nurse and Hospital Review* 16, no. 3 (March 1896): 125–27.

59. Taylor, "Obstetric Nursing," 128–29.

60. Gretchen Condram, "Changing Patterns of Epidemic Disease in New York City," in *Hives of Sickness: Public Health and Epidemics in New York City*, ed. David Rosner (New Jersey: Rutgers University Press, 1995), 27–41 (quote p. 30).

61. Markel, *Quarantine*.

62. Markel, *Quarantine*, 15–25.

63. Markel, *Quarantine*, 25–27.

64. Markel, *Quarantine*, 55–57.

65. Markel, *Quarantine*, 93.

66. Markel, *Quarantine*, 93.

67. Markel, *Quarantine*, 101–2.

68. Keeling, *Nursing and the Privilege of Prescription*. See also Markel, "'Knocking out Cholera," 420–57.

69. Markel, *Quarantine*, 93.

70. "Fire on Ellis Island," *New York Tribune*, June 15, 1897.

71. "Three Quarter Million Loss: Additional Particulars of the Fire on Ellis Island," *Wichita Daily Eagle*, June 16, 1897. Miss Holz is referred to as Miss Boltz in this article and no first name is given.

72. "Scenes of Terror at Ellis Island," *Brooklyn Eagle*, June 15, 1897.

73. "Three Quarter Million Loss."

74. "Three Quarter Million Loss."

75. "Fire on Ellis Island," *New York Times*, June 15, 1897. See also "Fire on Ellis Island," *New York Tribune*, June 15, 1897.

76. "Three Quarter Million Loss."

77. Stakely, *Cultural Landscape Report*, 29.

78. "Caring for the Immigrants: New Arrangements in Consequence of Yesterday Morning's Fire on Ellis Island," *New York Times*, June 16, 1897.

79. Margaret V. Daly, "Nursing at Ellis Island: A Memoir," unpublished manuscript, n.d., typescript. Manuscript initially accessed October 16, 2019 from *Bishop Hobbies*, https://www.bishophobbies.com/category/other-stuff/margaret-v-daly/. The manuscript is ten typed pages with five additional pages of typed notes with Margaret V. Daly listed as author. Mr. Floyd Paul Bishop, great-grandnephew of Ms. Daly, posted the scanned pages online after discovering them in a box given to him by his mother, Ms. Helen Ramona Johnson. Determining the authenticity of the pages involved triangulation with multiple sources. After discovering them online, Dr. Hehman initiated direct contact with Mr. Bishop and his wife Nina Bishop, who furnished genealogy records demonstrating that Ms. Johnson is the granddaughter of Ms. Jennie Daly, sister of Margaret Daly, as well as copies of Margaret Daly's death record and local obituaries. Using the additional data and with the family's permission, Dr. Hehman requested Ms. Daly's federal employment record from the Official Personnel Files office at the National Archives in St. Louis. Content, dates, and a significant number of unique details were corroborated in both the manuscript pages and Ms. Daly's employment records. Data from the 1930 US Census also show Margaret V. Daly, age fifty-two, boarding at the United States Marine Hospital at Ellis Island with her occupation listed as "Nurse." Final verification efforts included multiple consultations with coauthor Dr. Arlene Keeling and other Ellis Island experts, who agree that the available primary and secondary source material substantiate the validity of the manuscript contents. While the exact date of the manuscript is unknown, it was likely written in 1936 once Ms. Daly retired from duty at Ellis Island after being diagnosed with tuberculosis; she died just a few months later at Seton Hospital, a New York sanatorium, where she had moved to convalesce following her diagnosis.

CHAPTER 2

1. Margaret V. Daly, "Nursing at Ellis Island: A Memoir," unpublished manuscript, n.d., typescript, 1, available at *Bishop Hobbies*, accessed October 16, 2019, https://www.bishophobbies.com/category/other-stuff/margaret-v-daly/.

2. Daly, "Nursing at Ellis Island," 1.

3. Daly, "Nursing at Ellis Island," 1; "Day force" ferry information from William Williams, "Organization of the U.S. Immigrant Station at Ellis Island, New York, Together with a Brief Description of the Work Done in Each of Its Divisions," as cited in Harlan D. Unrau, *Historic Resource Study, Ellis Island, Statue of Liberty National Monument New York–New Jersey*, vol. 2 (Denver: US Department of the Interior National Park Service, 1984), 358.

4. Emma Lazarus, "The New Colossus," 1883, Library of Congress, https://www.loc .gov/exhibits/haventohome/images/hh0041s.jpg.

5. Sir Auckland Geddes, "Dispatch from H. M. Ambassador at Washington Reporting on Conditions at Ellis Island Immigration Station," 1923, as cited in Unrau, *Historic Resource Study*, vol. 2, 569.

6. Lori Conway, *Forgotten Ellis Island: The Extraordinary Story of America's Immigrant Hospital* (New York: HarperCollins, 2007), 6.

7. Margaret V. Daly, "Untitled notes," unpublished manuscript, n.d., typescript, 2, available at *Bishop Hobbies*, accessed October 16, 2019, https://www.bishophobbies .com/category/other-stuff/margaret-v-daly/2. These are five pages of untitled, undated, typed notes, found by Daly's great-grandnephew Paul Bishop alongside Daly's unpublished memoir, "Nursing at Ellis Island: A Memoir." The untitled notes contain Daly's random thoughts and memories about her experience working on Ellis Island from 1902 through her retirement in 1936.

8. Daly, "Nursing at Ellis Island," 1.

9. Milton H. Foster, "A General Hospital for All Nations," *Survey* 33, no. 22 (February 1915): 588.

10. Michelle C. Hehman, "Nurses, Science, and the Growth of Hospitals," in *History of Professional Nursing in the United States: Toward a Culture of Health*, ed. Arlene W. Keeling, Michelle C. Hehman, and John C. Kirchgessner (New York: Springer, 2018), 156–85.

11. Foster, "General Hospital for All Nations," 588.

12. Conway, *Forgotten Ellis Island*, 72–79.

13. Harlan D. Unrau, *Historic Structure Report, Ellis Island-Statue of Liberty National Monument* (Denver, CO: US Department of the Interior National Park Service, 1981), 424.

14. Lucy Minnigerode, "The Public Health Service Nursing Corps," *Public Health Reports* 42, no. 27 (1927): 1797–800.

15. In 1912 the United States Public Health and Marine Hospital Service was renamed a final time, to the United States Public Health Service.

16. Grover A. Kempf, oral history interview with Elizabeth Yew, September 10–11, 1977, courtesy the Statue of Liberty–Ellis Island Foundation, Inc., Ellis Island Oral History Project.

17. Clara Weeks-Shaw, *A Textbook of Nursing: For the Use of Training Schools, Families, and Private Students* (New York: D. Appleton, 1906), 19.

18. Isabel Adams Hampton, *Nursing, Its Principles and Its Practice: For Hospital and Private Use* (Philadelphia: W. B. Saunders, 1893), 44.

19. Weeks-Shaw, *Textbook of Nursing*, 19.

20. Weeks-Shaw, *Textbook of Nursing*, 6.

21. Treasury Department, *Regulations Governing the Uniforms of Officers and Employees of the United States Public Health Service* (Washington, DC: Government Printing Office, 1914), 33.

22. Treasury Department, *Regulations Governing the Uniforms*, 34.

23. Michelle C. Hehman, "The Rise of a Profession, 1873–1901," in Keeling, Hehman, and Kirchgessner, *History of Professional Nursing in the United States*, 44–71.

24. United States Treasury Department, *Regulations for the Government of the United States Public Health Service* (Washington, DC: Government Printing Office, 1913), 24.

25. Using available photographs of USPHS nurses between 1902 and 1916, all nurses pictured are White. Census data corroborates that all nurses on Ellis Island were White.

26. Mable K. Staupers, *No Time for Prejudice: A Story of the Integration of Negroes in Nursing in the United States* (New York: Macmillan, 1961), 17.

27. Josephine Friedman Lutomski, oral history interview with Edward Applebome, February 10, 1986, courtesy the Statue of Liberty–Ellis Island Foundation, Inc., Ellis Island Oral History Project.

28. Daly, "Untitled notes," 3.

29. US Congress, *An Act in Amendment to the Various Acts Relative to Immigration and the Importation of Aliens under Contract or Agreement to Perform Labor (1891 Immigration Act)*, 51st Congress, Session 2, chap. 551, 26 Statutes-at-Large 1084, March 3, 1891.

30. Foster, "General Hospital for All Nations."

31. The immigrant inspection process and USPHS procedures have been extensively detailed in a number of primary and secondary sources. See Bureau of Public Health and Marine Hospital Service, *Medical Inspection of Immigrants* (Washington, DC: Government Printing Office, 1903); United States Public Health Service, *Miscellaneous Publication no. 5: Regulations Governing the Medical Inspection of Aliens* (Washington, DC: Government Printing Office, 1917); E. H. Mullan, "Mental Examination of Immigrants: Administration and Line Inspection at Ellis Island," *Public Health Reports* 32 (May 18, 1917): 733–46; Alfred C. Reed, "Going through Ellis Island," *Popular Science Monthly* 82 (January 1913): 5–18; Howard Markel and Alexandra Minna Stern, "Which Face? Whose Nation? Immigration, Public Health, and the Construction of Disease at America's Ports and Borders, 1891–1928," *American Behavioral Scientist* 42 (June/July 1999): 1314–31; Elizabeth Yew, "Medical Inspection of Immigrants at Ellis Island, 1891–1924," *Bulletin of the New York Academy of Medicine* 55 (June 1980): 488–510; Anne-Emanuelle Birn, "Six Seconds per Eyelid: The Medical Inspection of Immigrants at Ellis Island, 1892–1914," *Dynamis* 17 (1997): 281–316; Conway, *Forgotten Ellis Island*, 32–69; Thomas M. Pitkin, *Keepers of the Gate: A History of Ellis Island* (New York: New York University Press, 1975), 68–70; Unrau, *Historic Resource Study*, vol. 2, 575–706.

32. The medical examination process at Ellis Island became known as the "Line" and USPHS physicians refer to their assignments in this capacity as "line duty" in memoirs and oral histories. See Mullan, "Mental Examination of Immigrants," 733–46;

Ralph Chester Williams, *The United States Public Health Service, 1798–1950* (Richmond: Whitney & Shepperson, 1951), 10 and 100; and T. Bruce H. Anderson, oral history interview by Elizabeth Yew, September 22, 1977, courtesy the Statue of Liberty–Ellis Island Foundation, Inc., Ellis Island Oral History Project. Anderson was a USPHS physician assigned to duty on Ellis Island beginning in 1919.

33. Frederick J. Haskin, *The Immigrant: An Asset and a Liability* (New York: Frederick A. Stokes, 1913), 27–34.

34. Mullan, "Mental Examination of Immigrants," 736.

35. Markel and Stern, "Which Face? Whose Nation?" 1318; Mullan, "Mental Examination of Immigrants," 736.

36. Barry Moreno, *Illustrated Encyclopedia of Ellis Island* (Westport, CT: Greenwood Press, 2004), 64.

37. Kempf interview.

38. Treasury Department, *Book of Instructions for the Medical Inspection of Immigrants* (Washington, DC: Government Printing Office, 1903), 6.

39. Emmanuel Steen, oral history interview with Paul Sigrist, March 22, 1991, courtesy the Statue of Liberty-Ellis Island Foundation, Inc., Ellis Island Oral History Project.

40. Alison Bateman-House and Amy Fairchild, "Medical Examination of Immigrants at Ellis Island," *Virtual Mentor* 10, no. 4 (2008): 235–41.

41. Bureau of Public Health, *Medical Inspection of Immigrants*, 6.

42. H. D. Geddings, "Investigations of Medical Policies, Procedures, and Personnel Practices at Ellis Island," report to the surgeon general, November 16, 1906, as cited in Unrau, *Historic Resource Study*, vol. 2, 665.

43. Weeks-Shaw, *Textbook of Nursing*, 112.

44. Mullan, "Mental Examination of Immigrants," 736.

45. Daly, "Untitled notes," 3.

46. Daly, "Untitled notes," 3.

47. Weeks-Shaw, *Textbook of Nursing*, 76.

48. Lutomski interview. A contract with the Troy Laundry Machinery Company indicates that laundry machinery was installed in 1901 in the hospital outbuilding on Island 2, as cited in Unrau, *Historic Structure Report*, 439.

49. Weeks-Shaw, *Textbook of Nursing*, 112–14.

50. Weeks-Shaw, *Textbook of Nursing*, 110.

51. Lavinia L. Dock, *Textbook of Materia Medica for Nurses*, 4th ed. (New York: G. P. Putnam's Sons, 1905).

52. Weeks-Shaw, *Textbook of Nursing*, 154–58.

53. Anna Caroline Maxwell and Amy Elizabeth Pope, *Practical Nursing: A Text-Book for Nurses* (New York: G. P. Putnam's Sons, 1907), 372.

54. Maxwell and Pope, *Practical Nursing*, 372.

55. Daly, "Nursing at Ellis Island," 2.

56. Daly, "Nursing at Ellis Island," 1–2.

57. See annual reports of the surgeon general of the United States from the years 1902 through 1917.

58. Daly, "Nursing at Ellis Island," 2.

59. Daly, "Nursing at Ellis Island," 1.

60. Daly, "Untitled notes," 2.

61. Hehman, "Nurses, Science, and the Growth of Hospitals," 54.

62. Treasury Department, *Regulations Governing the Hospitals and Relief Stations of the United States Public Health Service* (Washington, DC: Government Printing Office, 1920), 33.

63. Lavinia Dock, "The Relation of Training Schools to Hospitals," in *Nursing of the Sick, 1893, by Isabel A. Hampton and Others: Papers and Discussions from the International Congress of Charities, Correction and Philanthropy, Chicago, 1893* (New York: McGraw-Hill, 1949), 16.

64. Patricia D'Antonio, *American Nursing: A History of Knowledge, Authority, and the Meaning of Work* (Baltimore: Johns Hopkins University Press, 2010), 50.

65. W. C. Billings to US surgeon general, August 25, 1925; Official Personnel Folder (hereafter OPF) of Margaret Veronica Daly, courtesy the National Personnel Records Center at the National Archives, St. Louis (hereafter NPRC).

66. Unrau, *Historic Resource Study*, vol. 2, 724.

67. "Public Health Service Employees at Ellis Island: 1913," as cited in Unrau, *Historic Resource Study*, vol. 2, 713.

68. Billings to the surgeon general.

69. Daly, "Nursing at Ellis Island," 7.

70. Foster, "General Hospital for All Nations," 588.

71. J. E. Warper to the Secretary of the Treasury, February 11, 1925; OPF of Margaret Veronica Daly, courtesy the NPRC.

72. Reed, "Going through Ellis Island," 11.

73. Treasury Department, "Memorandum for Chief Medical Officer," February 4, 1925; OPF of Margaret Veronica Daly, courtesy the NPRC. The memorandum lists Ms. Daly's graduation date and program, as well as a detailed work history with the dates and names of every hospital she was affiliated with prior to her appointment on Ellis Island. Facilities included Roosevelt Hospital, Randall's Island Hospital, Mothers and Babies Hospital in New York, and the Contagious Disease Hospital at Hart's Island.

74. Daly, "Untitled notes," 5.

75. William Williams to the commissioner general of immigration, January 3, 1911; General Records of the Immigration and Naturalization Service, 1787–1993, Record Group 85 (hereafter RG 85); National Archives Building, Washington, DC (hereafter NAB).

76. Williams to the commissioner general.

77. Foster, "General Hospital for All Nations," 589.

78. Daly, "Untitled notes," 2.

79. John Henry Wilberding, oral history interview with Paul E. Sigrist Jr., May 11, 1998, courtesy the Statue of Liberty–Ellis Island Foundation, Inc., Ellis Island Oral History Project. Wilberding was a German immigrant who came through Ellis Island in 1928 as a six-year-old boy and was treated for measles in the Contagious Disease Hospital.

80. Daly, "Untitled notes," 4.

81. Wilberding interview.

82. Daly, "Untitled notes," 5.

83. Lutomski interview.

84. Daly, "Untitled notes," 5.

85. Terence V. Powderly, "Annual Report, Commissioner General of Immigration, Fiscal Year 1901," 38, as cited in Unrau, *Historic Structure Report*, 424.

86. Daly, "Nursing at Ellis Island," 2.

87. William Williams, *Annual Report of the Commissioner-General of Immigration for the Fiscal Year Ended June 30, 1903* (Washington, DC: Government Printing Office, 1903), 68.

88. Daly, "Nursing at Ellis Island," 2.

89. Unrau, *Historic Structure Report*, 459.

90. Daly, "Nursing at Ellis Island," 2.

91. William Williams, "Organization of the U.S. Immigration Station at Ellis Island, New York, Together with a Brief Description of the Work Done in Each of the Divisions," October 1903; General Immigration Files, RG 85, NAB.

92. Immigration Service, *Annual Report of the Superintendent of Immigration to the Secretary of the Treasury for the Fiscal Year Ended June 30, 1894* (Washington, DC: Government Printing Office, 1894), 24.

93. Daly, "Nursing on Ellis Island," 2.

94. J. G. Wilson, "Infectious Diseases of Children: A Study of 6,078 Cases among Immigrants with Special Reference to Cross Infection and Hospital Management," *Public Health Bulletin* 95 (October 1918): 8; US Bureau of the Census, *Bulletin 109: Mortality Statistics: 1910* (Washington, DC: Government Printing Office, 1912), 25–26.

95. Howard Markel and Alexandra Minna Stern, "The Foreignness of Germs: The Persistent Association of Immigrants and Disease in American Society," *Milbank Quarterly* 80, no. 4 (2002): 757–88.

96. Terence V. Powderly, "Immigration's Menace to National Health," *North American Review* 175, no. 548 (1902): 56–57; Foster, "General Hospital for All Nations," 588.

97. Assistant surgeon of the Public Health and Marine Hospital Service to the commissioner of immigration at Ellis Island, July 16, 1906; General Immigration Files, RG 85, NAB.

98. "Annual Report to the Commissioner of Immigration," July 16, 1906, General Immigration Files, RG 85, NAB. The "Summary of Hospital Transactions" lists the total number of immigrant patients sent to outside hospitals (Health Department hospitals, Long Island College Hospital, and St. Vincent's Hospital) as 2,551; the "Financial Statement: Medical Department" lists total costs for "the care and maintenance of

immigrant patients" at each hospital, as well as to ambulance contractor Michael Hassett for transportation and burial services for immigrants, at a grand total of $110,893.50.

99. Williams, *Annual Report, June 30, 1903*, 68.
100. Walter Wyman to commissioner-general of immigration, November 26, 1902, and White, Pettus, Vaughan, Geddings, and Rosenau to Surgeon General, November 6, 1902, General Immigration Files, RG 85, NAB; "Report of the Commissioner-General of Immigration, July 1, 1906," as cited in Unrau, *Historic Structure Report*, 515.
101. Daly, "Untitled notes," 2.
102. J. Tracy Stakely, *Cultural Landscape Report for Ellis Island, Statue of Liberty National Monument* (Brookline: Olmstead Center for Landscape Preservation, 2003), 51.
103. Chief Surgeon Stoner to Supervising Architect Taylor, February 15, 1906, as cited in Unrau, *Historic Structure Report*, 512.
104. Maxwell and Pope, *Practical Nursing*, 340.
105. Unrau, *Historic Structure Report*, 529–38.

CHAPTER 3

1. Margaret V. Daly, "Nursing at Ellis Island: A Memoir," unpublished manuscript, n.d., typescript, 2, available at *Bishop Hobbies*, accessed October 16, 2019, https://www.bishophobbies.com/category/other-stuff/margaret-v-daly/.
2. "Obituary, Margaret V. Daily," *Old Castle Garden* 6, no. 4 (December 1936): 99. The obituary describes Margaret as a "faithful member of the congregation all these years." Details of Margaret's church affiliation were confirmed by family members Paul and Nina Bishop.
3. Daly, "Nursing at Ellis Island," 2.
4. J. G. Wilson, "Infectious Diseases of Children: A Study of 6,078 Cases among Immigrants with Special Reference to Cross Infection and Hospital Management," *Public Health Bulletin* 95 (October 1918): 85–88.
5. Patricia D'Antonio, *American Nursing: A History of Knowledge, Authority, and the Meaning of Work* (Baltimore: Johns Hopkins University Press, 2010), 36.
6. Clara Weeks-Shaw, *A Textbook of Nursing: For the Use of Training Schools, Families, and Private Students* (New York: D. Appleton, 1885), 183.
7. "Instructions to Be Followed by Those Who Work in the Contagious Wards in the Contagious Disease Hospital," in Harlan D. Unrau, *Historic Resource Study, Ellis Island, Statue of Liberty National Monument New York–New Jersey*, vol. 2 (Denver: US Department of the Interior National Park Service, 1984), 727.
8. "Instructions to Be Followed," 727. The mattress autoclave on Island 3 (the same island housing the contagious disease hospital) can still be seen during the hard hat tour of the Ellis Island hospital facilities. An image and explanation of the machine can be found at https://www.nps.gov/media/photo/gallery-item.htm?id=378AC5EE-155D-451F-673B22210931AA50&gid=37de920f-155d-451f-67426c8113e9361f.
9. Wilson, "Infectious Diseases of Children," 85–86.

10. Wilson, "Infectious Diseases of Children," 86.

11. Wilson, "Infectious Diseases of Children," 7–8.

12. J. G. Wilson, "The Contagious Disease Hospital for Immigrants at Ellis Island," *Modern Hospital* 9, no. 5 (November 1917): 316.

13. Wilson, "Infectious Diseases of Children," 86–88.

14. "Memoranda Governing Admittance to Contagious Disease Hospital," in Unrau, *Historic Resource Study*, vol. 2, 726.

15. "Instructions to Be Followed," 727.

16. Wilson, "Infectious Diseases of Children," 85.

17. Wilson, "Contagious Disease Hospital," 316.

18. Wilson, "Contagious Disease Hospital," 313.

19. Wilson, "Infectious Diseases of Children," 8–9.

20. Wilson, "Contagious Disease Hospital," 313.

21. Incidence of cross-infection cited in Wilson, "Contagious Disease Hospital," 313; mortality statistics found in Wilson, "Infectious Diseases of Children," 12.

22. G. W. Stoner to Taylor, February 15, 1906, as cited in Harlan D. Unrau, *Historic Structure Report: Statue of Liberty Ellis Island* (Denver: United States Department of the Interior, 1981), 512.

23. Wilson, "Infectious Diseases of Children," 8–9.

24. William Butler, "The Fatality Rate of Measles: A Study of Its Trend in Time," *Journal of the Royal Statistical Society* 108, parts 3–4 (1945): 260.

25. Milton H. Foster, "A General Hospital for All Nations," *Survey* 33, no. 22 (February 1915): 589.

26. Frederick S. Crum, "A Statistical Study of Measles," *American Journal of Public Health* 4, no. 4 (April 1914): 289.

27. Wilson, "Infectious Diseases of Children," 13–16.

28. Wilson, "Infectious Diseases of Children," 50.

29. Admission frequencies for measles in the contagious disease hospital between 1912 and 1916 consistently show spikes in winter months, with December 1914 as the busiest month on record, see Wilson, "Infectious Diseases of Children," 29.

30. Daly, "Nursing at Ellis Island," 7.

31. Unrau, *Historic Resource Study*, vol. 2, 538.

32. Treatment of measles described in Anna Caroline Maxwell and Amy Elizabeth Pope, *Practical Nursing: A Text-Book for Nurses* (New York: G. P. Putnam's Sons, 1907), 362–64; and W. G. Stimpson, *Prevention of Disease and Care of the Sick: How to Keep Well and What to Do in Case of Sudden Illness* (Washington, DC: Government Printing Office, 1918), 123–25.

33. Stimpson, *Prevention of Disease*, 124.

34. Treatment of measles described in Maxwell, *Practical Nursing*, 362–64; and in Stimpson, *Prevention of Disease*, 123–25.

35. "Bill of Fare for the Immigrant Dining Room," Bob Hope Memorial Library, Archives and Special Collections, National Park Service at Ellis Island.

36. John Henry Wilberding, oral history interview by Paul E. Sigrist Jr., May 11, 1998, courtesy the Statue of Liberty–Ellis Island Foundation, Inc., Ellis Island Oral History Project.

37. Thomas Allan, oral history interview by Jean Kolva, July 16, 1984, courtesy the Statue of Liberty–Ellis Island Foundation, Inc., Ellis Island Oral History Project.

38. Josephine Friedman Lutomski, oral history interview by Edward Applebome, February 10, 1986, courtesy the Statue of Liberty–Ellis Island Foundation, Inc., Ellis Island Oral History Project.

39. Wilson, "Infectious Diseases of Children," 88.

40. Wilson, "Infectious Diseases of Children," 88–89.

41. Wilson, "Infectious Diseases of Children," 89.

42. Wilson, "Infectious Diseases of Children," 29.

43. Daly, "Nursing at Ellis Island," 9.

44. Terence V. Powderly, "Immigration's Menace to the National Health," *North American Review* 175, no. 548 (July 1902): 55.

45. Amy Fairchild, *Science at the Borders: Immigrant Medical Inspection and the Shaping of the Modern Industrial Labor Force* (Baltimore: Johns Hopkins University Press, 2003), 40.

46. Henry W. Dearborn, *Diseases of the Skin: Their Symptomatology, Etiology and Diagnosis with Special Reference to Principles of Treatment Including Full Indications for Drug Remedies*, 2nd ed. (New York: Boericke and Runyou, 1906), 298.

47. Powderly, "Immigration's Menace to the National Health," 59–60.

48. Unrau, *Historic Structure Report*, 538.

49. Dearborn, *Diseases of the Skin*, 301.

50. Dearborn, *Diseases of the Skin*, 301.

51. Dr. Carl Ramus, Acting Chief Medical Officer, as cited in Lorie Conway, *Forgotten Ellis Island: The Extraordinary Story of America's Immigrant Hospital* (New York: Smithsonian Books, 2007), 94.

52. Dearborn, *Diseases of the Skin*, 301.

53. T. Clark and J. W. Schereschewsky, *Trachoma: Its Character and Effects* (Washington, DC: Government Printing Office, 1907), 3.

54. Howard Markel, "'The Eyes Have It': Trachoma, the Perception of Disease, the United States Public Health Service, and the American Jewish Immigration Experience," *Bulletin of the History of Medicine* 74, no. 3 (2000): 533; Clark and Schereschewsky, *Trachoma*, 4.

55. Information compiled from Annual Reports of the US commissioner-general of immigration, 1900–1920, as cited in Markel, "The Eyes Have It," 552.

56. Clark and Schereschewsky, *Trachoma*, 20.

57. Clark and Schereschewsky, *Trachoma*, 30.

58. Minnie Goodnow, *First-Year Nursing: A Text-Book for Pupils during Their First Year of Hospital Work* (Philadelphia: W. B. Saunders, 1916), 293–94.

59. Clark and Schereschewsky, *Trachoma*, 30–31.

60. Details of the USPHS trachoma treatment regimen can be found in Clark and Schereschewsky, *Trachoma*, 30–32.

61. Josephine Gazieri Calloway, oral history interview by Judith Hartman, June 17, 1986, courtesy the Statue of Liberty–Ellis Island Foundation, Inc., Ellis Island Oral History Project.

62. Calloway interview.

63. Daly, "Nursing at Ellis Island," 8.

64. Gertrude Slaughter, "America's Front Door," *Hygeia* 11 (January 1933): 11–14.

65. Grover A. Kempf, oral history interview with Elizabeth Yew, September 10–11, 1977, courtesy the Statue of Liberty-Ellis Island Foundation, Inc., Ellis Island Oral History Project.

66. Conway, *Forgotten Ellis Island*, 6.

67. Arlene Keeling, "Reflections on Immigration: The Nurses of Ellis Island," *Windows in Time: The Newsletter of the UVA Eleanor Crowder Bjoring Center for Nursing Historical Inquiry*, 22, no. 2 (October 2014): 2.

68. Conway, *Forgotten Ellis Island*, 109.

69. S. J. Williams to Rupert Blue, October 29, 1913; Central Files 1897–1923, box 023, Records of the Public Health Service, Record Group 90 (hereafter RG 90), National Archives at College Park, MD (hereafter NACP).

70. Surgeon General Rupert Blue to S. J. Williams, November 10, 1913; Central Files 1897–1923, box 023, RG90, NACP.

71. Daly, "Nursing at Ellis Island," 1.

72. Daly, "Nursing at Ellis Island," 10.

73. Daly, "Nursing at Ellis Island," 2.

74. "Report of the Commissioner General of Immigration," in *Third Annual Report of the Secretary of Labor, Fiscal Year Ended June 30, 1915* (Washington, DC: Government Printing Office, 1915), 59.

75. "Reports of the Commissioner General of Immigration," fiscal years 1914–1917, as cited in Unrau, *Historic Resource Study*, vol. 2, 734.

76. Daly, "Nursing at Ellis Island," 2.

77. Daly, "Nursing at Ellis Island," 2.

CHAPTER 4

1. Margaret V. Daly, "Nursing at Ellis Island: A Memoir," unpublished manuscript, n.d., typescript, 1, available at *Bishop Hobbies*, accessed October 16, 2019, https://www.bishophobbies.com/category/other-stuff/margaret-v-daly/.

2. Bernard Marinbach, *Galveston: Ellis Island of the West* (Albany: SUNY Press, 1983).

3. Daly, "Nursing at Ellis Island," 2–3.

4. Susan Reverby, *Ordered to Care: The Dilemma of American Nursing, 1850–1945* (Cambridge: Cambridge University Press, 1987).

5. Daly, "Nursing at Ellis Island," 2–3.

6. Daly, "Nursing at Ellis Island," 3.

7. Jane Delano, "The Need for Increased Enrollment," *American Journal of Nursing* 17, no. 11 (August 1917): 1092–97.

8. Portia Kernodle, *Red Cross Nurse in Action* (New York: Harper and Brothers, 1949), 108–9. In order to enlist, the nurses had to meet specific criteria. In 1917, US Army nurses had to be US citizens between the ages of twenty-five and thirty-five years. They also had to be single, White, and female. In addition, they had to be graduates of training schools of nursing linked with hospitals of more than fifty beds. Clearly, the criteria discriminated against male nurses and Blacks.

9. Arlene W. Keeling, "Nurses in the News: The Great War and Pandemic Influenza 1914–1919," in *History of Professional Nursing in the United States*, ed. Arlene Keeling, Michelle Hehman, and John Kirchgessner (New York: Springer 2018), 189–90.

10. Army nurses were part of the American Red Cross at this time.

11. L. L. Williams to the surgeon general, United States Public Health Service, August 2, 1915, Central File, 1897–1923, box 037, Records of the Public Health Service, Record Group 90 (hereafter RG 90), National Archives at College Park, MD (hereafter NACP).

12. Lavinia Dock, Sarah Pickett, Clara Noyes, Fannie Clement, Elizabeth Fox, and Ann Van Meter, *History of American Red Cross Nursing* (New York: Macmillan, 1922), 416. Following her graduation from the Waldeck Hospital Training School in San Francisco, Mury worked in several US and Philippine hospitals and subsequently served three years in the Navy Nurse Corps. In July 1916 she was transferred to the Army Nurse Corps where she worked as assistant superintendent. She also served in the US surgeon general's Office.

13. Dock et al., *History of American Red Cross Nursing*, 416.

14. Edith Mury, quoted in Dock et al., *History of American Red Cross Nursing*, 417.

15. Dock et al., *History of American Red Cross Nursing*, 417.

16. Mury, quoted in Dock et al., *History of American Red Cross Nursing*, 416.

17. Dock et al., *History of American Red Cross Nursing*, 416.

18. Dock et al. *History of American Red Cross Nursing*, 416.

19. *History of Base Hospital #20 Organized by the University of Pennsylvania* (Philadelphia: E. A. Wright, 1920), 29.

20. Dock et al., *History of American Red Cross Nursing*, 416.

21. Dock et al., *History of American Red Cross Nursing*, 417.

22. Mury, quoted in Dock et al., *History of American Red Cross Nursing*, 417.

23. Dock et al., *History of American Red Cross Nursing*, 494.

24. Sarah Parsons, *History of Massachusetts General Hospital (MGH Training School) for Nurses* (Boston: Whitcomb and Barrows, 1922), 48.

25. Clara Noyes, telegram to Sarah E. Parsons, May 22, 1917, Massachusetts General Hospital School of Nursing Archives. See https://archive.org.

26. Sarah Parsons, photo of Diary page 1917, in Massachusetts General Hospital Nursing History Committee, "MGH Nurses Serve in WWI before They Have Right to Vote," *Caring Headlines* (May 4, 2017): 5.

27. Sarah Parsons, "The Nurse's Point of View," in *History of Base Hospital 6*, ed. George Clymer, Ralph Heard, George Leland, James Means, and Paul White (Boston: n.p., 1924), 51.

28. Dock et al., *History of American Red Cross Nursing*, 417.

29. Clymer et al., *History of Base Hospital 6*, 53.

30. Dock et al., *History of American Red Cross Nursing*, 417.

31. Clymer et al., *History of Base Hospital 6*, 52.

32. Parsons, "Nurse's Point of View," 53.

33. Dock et al., *History of American Red Cross Nursing*, 369.

34. Delano, "The Need for Increased Enrollment," 1092–97.

35. "Mobilization Papers for E. Blanche Augustine, from the United States Army Nurse Corps, War Department, Office of the Surgeon General," Digital Collections, Robert L. Brown History of Medicine Collection, University of Buffalo Library, https://digital .lib.buffalo.edu/items/show 93213.

36. Elsie Blanche Augustine, chap. 2 in *Diary of a U.S. Army Nurse in the Great War*, September 1, 1917, 16–40 (quote p. 16), Digital Collections, Robert L. Brown History of Medicine Collection, University of Buffalo Library, https://digital.lib.buffalo.edu /items/show 93213.

37. Augustine, chap. 2 in *Diary of a U.S. Army Nurse*.

38. Mury, quoted in Dock et al., *History of American Red Cross Nursing*, 419.

39. Augustine, chap. 2 in *Diary of a U.S. Army Nurse*, 33.

40. Dock et al., *History of American Red Cross Nursing*, 420.

41. Clara Noyes quoted in Dock et al., *History of American Red Cross Nursing*, 371.

42. Alma Wooley, "A Hoosier Nurse in France: The World War I Diary of Maude Francis Essig," *Indiana Magazine of History* 82, no. 1 (March 1986): 37–68.

43. Dora Thompson, "Important Instructions to Members of the ANC Designated for Service Abroad," *American Journal of Nursing* 18, no. 4 (January 1918): 335–37 (quote p. 335).

44. Augustine, *Diary of a U.S. Army Nurse*, November 21–22, 1917, pp. 35–37.

45. Augustine, *Diary of a U.S. Army Nurse*, November 22, 1917, p. 37.

46. Arlene Keeling, "Nursing in the News," 191.

47. Edmond Pitts, ed., *Base Hospital 34 in the World War* (Philadelphia: Lyon and Armor Printers, 1922), 30–136, available at https://www.collections.nlm.nih.gov /14230650R.

48. Dock et al., *History of American Red Cross Nursing*, 424.

49. *History of Base Hospital #20*, 29, National Library of Medicine, Digital Collections, accessed May 18, 2024, http://resource.nlm.nih.gov/9110805?.

50. Flora Graham, Jean Haviland, and Glenna Bigelow, "Ellis Island from Three Points of View," *American Journal of Nursing* 18, no. 8 (May 1918): 613–22 (quote p. 615).

51. Dock et al., *History of American Red Cross Nursing*, 417–20.

52. Glenna Bigelow, February 22, 1918, diary entry, quoted in Graham, Haviland, and Bigelow, "Ellis Island," 620.

53. Emma E. Weaver, *Journal of E. Elizabeth Weaver, Army Nurse Corps WW I*, February 27, 1918, https://www.armyheritage.org/soldier-stories-information/emma-elizabeth -weaver/. See also Christine Hallet, *Veiled Warriors: Allied Nurses of the First World War* (Oxford: Oxford University Press, 2014).

54. Parsons, "Nurse's Point of View," 53.

55. Graham, Haviland, and Bigelow, "Ellis Island," 620.

56. Dock et al., *History of American Red Cross Nursing*, 418.

57. Dock et al., *History of American Red Cross Nursing*, 417. See also Weaver, *Journal*, February 27, 1918.

58. Weaver, *Journal*, February 27, 1918.

59. T. Bruce Anderson, oral history interview with Paul Siegrist, September 22, 1977, courtesy the Statue of Liberty–Ellis Island Foundation, Inc., Ellis Island Oral History Project. Anderson was a USPHS physician stationed on Ellis Island in 1918.

60. Weaver, *Journal*, February 1918, 5.

61. Mury, quoted in Dock et al., *History of American Red Cross Nursing*, 419.

62. Bigelow, quoted in Dock et al., *History of American Red Cross Nursing*, 424.

63. Daly, "Nursing at Ellis Island," 3.

64. Torri Brouhard and Jim Peskin, "Ellis Island and the Great Spanish Flu," *Archivist* 49, no. 1–2 (May 2020): 1–20.

65. Surgeon J. W. Kerr, *Report*, July 17, 1918: 1–2, Central file, 1897–1923, box 037, RG90, NACP. In early April 1918, the Army Nurse Corps requisitioned a chain of twenty hotels in Manhattan as temporary housing for nurses before deployment overseas. The Holly Hotel on Washington Square West served as nursing headquarters.

66. Weaver, *Journal*, March 1–17, 1918. See also Dock et al., *History of American Red Cross Nursing*, 506; and *History of Base Hospital #20*.

67. Weaver, *Journal*, March 1–17, 1918.

68. Weaver, *Journal*, March 1–17, 1918.

69. Anderson interview.

70. Carol R. Byerly, *Fever of War: The Influenza Epidemic in the U.S. Army during World War I* (New York: New York University Press, 2005).

71. *The Pill Box: Newsletter of the U.S.A. Debarkation Hospital Number One, Ellis Island* (Ellis Island: The Medical and Quartermaster Detachments of Debarkation Hospital #1 publishers, August 31, 1918), 1.

72. Barry Kaufman, "Reading's Unsung Heroines: The Women of World War I," *History Review of Berks County* (Spring 2010): 75–80.

73. Chief Medical Officer, Ellis Island (name illegible), *Correspondence to the Surgeon General, USPHS* (9 July 1919): 1–2; Unrau Papers, box 8, Archives and Special Collections, Bob Hope Memorial Library, National Park Service at Ellis Island.

74. Chief Medical Officer to Surgeon General, 2.

75. Daly, "Nursing at Ellis Island," 7.

76. J. W. Kerr, Chief Medical Officer George W. Stoner to USPHS surgeon general, Washington, DC, July 5, 1919, Central file 1897–1923, RG 90, NACP.

77. Daly, "Nursing at Ellis Island," 7.

78. Daly, "Nursing at Ellis Island," 7.

CHAPTER 5

1.   J. W. Kerr, assistant surgeon general to US surgeon general, April 21, 1921, Unrau Papers, box 8, series 2, folder 113, Bob Hope Memorial Library, Archives and Special Collections, National Park Service at Ellis Island (hereafter cited as BHML-EI).

2.   Josephine Friedman Lutomski, oral history interview by Edward Applebome, February 10, 1986, courtesy the Statue of Liberty–Ellis Island Foundation, Inc., Ellis Island Oral History Project.

3.   W. G. Stimpson, *Prevention of Disease and Care of the Sick: How to Keep Well and What to Do in Case of Sudden Illness* (Washington, DC: Government Printing Office, 1919), 169.

4.   A list of all USPHS staff members stationed on Ellis Island is found in "Monthly Personnel Report: United States Public Health Service, U.S. Marine Hospital #43, Ellis Island, N.Y., March 1923," Unrau Papers, box 8, series IV, folder 113, BHML-EI.

5.   J. Tracy Stakely, *Cultural Landscape Report for Ellis Island, Statue of Liberty National Monument* (Brookline, MA: Olmstead Center for Landscape Preservation, 2003), 65.

6.   The hospitals on Ellis Island were returned to the Bureau of Immigration by the military on July 1, 1919, and were then officially transferred to the USPHS on September 1, 1919. At this point both hospital complexes were renamed United States Public Health Service Marine Hospital No. 43. See *Annual Report of the Surgeon General of the Public Health Service of the United States for the Fiscal Year 1920* (Washington, DC: Government Printing Office, 1920), 235.

7.   J. W. Kerr to the surgeon general of the USPHS, June 18, 1919, Central Files, 1897–1923, Records of the Public Health Service, Record Group 90 (hereafter RG 90), National Archives at College Park, MD (hereafter NACP).

8.   "Hospital Care of Aliens and a General Summary of the Medical Examination of Aliens, 1931," Central Files, 1897–1923, RG90, NACP.

9.   According to structural and construction records completed after 1920, the operating room and the chief nurse's quarters and bathroom were located on the third floor of the original hospital building on Island 2. See Harlan D. Unrau, *Historic Structure Report, Ellis Island–Statue of Liberty National Monument* (Denver: US Department of the Interior National Park Service, 1981), 480.

10. "Procedures to Be Followed in Operating Room, 1922–24," in Harlan D. Unrau, *Historic Resource Study, Ellis Island, Statue of Liberty National Monument New York–New Jersey*, vol. 2 (Denver: US Department of the Interior National Park Service, 1984), 729.

11. John Shaw Billings, "Medical Progress," *Medical News* 58 (1891): 669.

12. Michelle C. Hehman, "Nurses, Science, and the Growth of Hospitals," in *History of Professional Nursing in the United States: Toward a Culture of Health*, ed. Arlene W. Keeling, Michelle C. Hehman, and John C. Kirchgessner (New York: Springer, 2018), 164–67.

13. Atul Gawande, "Two Hundred Years of Surgery," *New England Journal of Medicine* 366 (2012): 1718–19.

14. Lindsey Fitzharris, *The Butchering Art: Joseph Lister's Quest to Transform the Grisly World of Victorian Medicine* (New York: Scientific American, 2017), 17.

15. See Fitzharris, *Butchering Art*, 17; and Hehman, "Nurses, Science, and the Growth of Hospitals," 164–67.

16. Justin Barr, Leopoldo C. Cancio, David J. Smith, Matthew J. Bradley, and Eric A. Alster, "From Trench to Bedside: Military Surgery during World War I upon Its Centennial," *Military Medicine* 184 (2019): 216.

17. Kim Pelis, "Taking Credit: The Canadian Army Medical Corps and the British Conversion to Blood Transfusion in WWI," *Journal of the History of Medicine and Allied Sciences* 56, no. 3 (July 2001): 238–77.

18. A. A. Martin, *A Surgeon in Khaki* (London: Edward Arnold, 1915), as cited in Barr et al., "From Trench to Bedside," 216.

19. See Christine E. Hallett, *Containing Trauma: Nursing in the First World War* (Manchester, UK: Manchester University Press, 2010); and Barr et al., "From Trench to Bedside," 214–20.

20. Hehman, "Nurses, Science, and the Growth of Hospitals," 164–67.

21. Leila Clark Woodbury, "Surgical Nursing," *American Journal of Nursing* 3, no. 9 (June 1903): 688–89.

22. Emma L. Colebourn is listed as "Nurse, Oper. room" in the Monthly Personnel Report, March 1924, sheet four, in "Synopsis for the Guidance of Hospital Inspectors, U.S. Marine Hospital #43, Ellis Island, New York," Unrau Papers, box 7, series IV, folder 111, BHML EI.

23. Margaret V. Daly, "Nursing at Ellis Island: A Memoir," unpublished manuscript, n.d., typescript, 8, available at *Bishop Hobbies*, accessed October 16, 2019, https://www.bishophobbies.com/category/other-stuff/margaret-v-daly/.

24. Daly, "Nursing at Ellis Island," 8.

25. Daly, "Nursing at Ellis Island," 8.

26. See "Synopsis for the Guidance of Hospital Inspectors: U.S. Marine Hospital #43, Ellis Island, N.Y. 1922–1924," Unrau Papers, box 8, series IV, folders 111–13, BHML-EI.

27. "Procedures to Be Followed," 728.

28. "Procedures to Be Followed," 728.

29. "Procedures to Be Followed," 728.

30. For names of surgical team, see C. K. Haskell, "Synopsis for the Guidance of Hospital Inspectors: U.S. Marine Hospital #43, Ellis Island, N.Y., April 19–23, 1923," Unrau Papers, box 8, series IV, folder 113, BHML-EI. Margaret Daly highlighted her nine years of experience in the operating room at Ellis Island in the form "United States Civil Service Commission, Graduate Nurse Examination," Official Personnel Folder (hereafter OPF) of Margaret Veronica Daly, courtesy the National Personnel Records Center at the National Archives, St. Louis (hereafter NPRC).

31. "Procedures to Be Followed," 728–29.

32. "Procedures to Be Followed," 729.

33. Robert H. M. Dawbarn, "Threatened Death during Major Anesthesia, with a Brief

Digression upon Shock," *Atlanta Medical and Surgical Journal* 14 (1897): 514.

34. "Procedures to Be Followed," 729.

35. Lutomski interview.

36. US Congress, *An Act to Regulate the Immigration of Aliens into the United States* (Immigration Act of 1907), 59th Congress, Session 2, chapter 1134, 34 Statutes-at-Large 898 (February 20, 1907).

37. See Howard Markel and Alexandra Minna Stern, "The Foreignness of Germs: The Persistent Association of Immigrants and Disease in American Society," *Milbank Quarterly* 80 (2002): 757–88; Stanley Coben, "A Study in Nativism: The American Red Scare of 1919–20," *Political Science Quarterly* 79 (1964): 52–75; and Michelle C. Hehman, "Nursing Care of Refugee Children: A Historical Perspective," *Pediatric Nursing* 48, no. 5 (October 2022): 215–21.

38. "To Halt the European Invasion," *Literary Digest* 67, no. 13 (December 25, 1920): 14.

39. US Congress, *An Act to Limit the Immigration of Aliens into the United States* (1921 Emergency Quota Law), 67th Congress, H.R. 4075, Pub.L. 67-5, Statute-at-Large 5 (May 19, 1921).

40. A. Warner Parker, "The Quota Provisions of the Immigration Act of 1924," *American Journal of International Law* 18 (1924): 737. Though the measure was regarded as "highly experimental," Congress renewed the act the following year, upholding the provisions until "a more scientific" and restrictive quota law was put in place.

41. Lorie Conway, *Forgotten Ellis Island: The Extraordinary Story of America's Immigrant Hospital* (New York: HarperCollins, 2007), 114–17. Conway describes the experience of Ormond McDermott at Ellis Island at length, including personal details gathered from McDermott's distant family in Australia.

42. Conway, *Forgotten Ellis Island*, 114.

43. "Methods of Medical Examination of Arriving Aliens," January 19, 1921, as cited in Unrau, *Historic Resource Study*, vol. 2, 626.

44. "Admission Chart, U.S. Public Health Service Hospital #43, Ellis Island, N.Y., McDermott, Ormond #10036, 2/25/21," Central File 1897–1923, box 023, RG 90, NACP.

45. "Admission Chart, U.S. Public Health Service Hospital #43, Ellis Island, N.Y."; and "Clinical Record: Nurse's Progress and Treatment Record, McDermott, Ormond #10036, from 02/26/1921 to 02/28/1921," Central File 1897–1923, box 104, RG 90, NACP.

46. "Admission Chart, U.S. Public Health Service Hospital #43, Ellis Island, N.Y."; and "Clinical Record: Nurse's Progress and Treatment Record."

47. Stimpson, *Prevention of Disease and Care of the Sick*, 126.

48. A. J. McLaughlin to US surgeon general Hugh S. Cumming, January 31, 1924, 6. The letter contains a ten-page report of the conditions and daily operations at Marine Hospital #43 (Ellis Island), including a description of each ward and its general use.

49. "Clinical Record: Ward Surgeon's Progress and Treatment Record, McDermott, Ormond #10036, from 02/26/1921 to 03/01/1921," and "Clinical Record: Nurse's Progress and Treatment Record," Central File 1897–1923, box 104, RG 90, NACP.

50. *Annual Report of the Surgeon General of the Public Health Service of the United States, for the Fiscal Year 1921* (Washington, DC: Government Printing Office, 1921), 248–49. The

volume of work performed by Ellis Island laboratory staff reflected this shift in medical practice; McDermott's throat culture was one of 5,184 processed in 1921, out of nearly 23,000 total laboratory specimens that year.

51. "Clinical Record: Nurse's Progress and Treatment Record."
52. "Clinical Record: Nurse's Progress and Treatment Record."
53. "Clinical Record: Ward Surgeon's Progress and Treatment Record."
54. "Clinical Record: Graphic Chart, Temperature, Etc., Feb 25–Mar.1," Central File, 1897–1923, box 104, RG90, NACP.
55. "Clinical Record: Ward Surgeon's Progress and Treatment Record."
56. "Clinical Record: Nurse's Progress and Treatment Record."
57. "Clinical Record: Brief, U.S. Public Health Service Hospital #43, Ellis Island, N.Y., Register No. 10036, McDermott, Ormond," Central File, 1897–1923, box 104, RG 90, NACP.
58. Haskell, "Synopsis for the Guidance of Hospital Inspectors."
59. Office of the Medical Officer in Charge, Ellis Island, N.Y. to Studebaker Corporation of America, March 8, 1921, Central File, 1897–1923, box 104, RG 90, NACP. The letter factually details McDermott's arrival to Ellis Island, dates of hospitalization, his cause of death, and a list of his belongings, including "1 British Passport."
60. *Regulations Governing the Medical Inspection of Aliens* (Washington, DC: Government Printing Office, 1917), 47.
61. *Regulations Governing the Medical Inspection of Aliens*, 42.
62. Surgeon General Hugh S. Cumming to Representative W. J. Graham, February 18, 1924, Unrau Papers, box 8, series IV, folder 113, BHML-EI.
63. USPHS surgeon A. J. MacLaughlin to Surgeon General Hugh S. Cumming, February 15, 1924, Unrau Papers, box 8, series IV, folder 113, BHML-EI. It had become "custom and procedure" for the Immigration Service to deport "pregnant women who show no signs of impending labor and who are able to travel," since transportation companies were required to maintain "doctors and hospital facilities on board ship."
64. MacLaughlin to Cumming, February 15, 1924.
65. Mrs. Hester to Representative W. J. Graham, February 10, 1924, Unrau Papers, box 8, series IV, folder 113, BHML-EI.
66. Hester to Graham, February 10, 1924.
67. Hester to Graham, February 10, 1924; and MacLaughlin to Cumming, February 15, 1924.
68. MacLaughlin to Cumming, February 15, 1924. This letter describes the course of Ruth Grahn's illness and hospitalization; and USPHS surgeon A. J. MacLaughlin, letter to Surgeon General Hugh S. Cumming, January 31, 1924, Unrau Papers, box 8, series IV, folder 113, BHML-EI. This letter describes the hospital operations on Ellis Island and gives a detailed description of each ward and the associated patients and diagnoses cared for in each one.
69. MacLaughlin to Cumming, February 15, 1924.
70. Stimpson, *Prevention of Disease and Care of the Sick*, 158.

71. MacLaughlin to Cumming, February 15, 1924.

72. Margaret V. Daly, "Untitled notes," unpublished manuscript, n.d., typescript, 2, available at *Bishop Hobbies*, accessed October 16, 2019, https://www.bishophobbies.com /category/other-stuff/margaret-v-daly/2.

73. Milton H. Foster, "A General Hospital for all Nations," *Survey* 33, no. 22 (February 1915): 588–90. Foster, a USPHS surgeon stationed on Ellis Island in the early twentieth century, explained that since the law did not consider that immigrants on Ellis Island had officially landed in the United States, infants born on Ellis Island did not receive automatic citizenship and were instead legally classified as though they had been "born on the high seas."

74. Daly, "Untitled notes," 2.

75. Daly, "Untitled notes," 2.

76. "Procedures to Be Followed," 729.

77. MacLaughlin to Cumming, February 15, 1924.

78. Surgeon General H. S. Cumming, letter to Honorable W. J. Graham, March 10, 1924, Unrau Papers, box 8, series IV, folder 113, BHML-EI.

79. MacLaughlin to Cumming, February 15, 1924.

80. Cumming to Graham, March 10, 1924.

81. See John W. Harris, "Influenza Occurring in Pregnant Women: A Statistical Study of Thirteen Hundred and Fifty Cases," *Journal of the American Medical Association* 72, no. 14 (1919): 978–80; and Paul Titus and J. M. Jamison, "Pregnancy Complicated by Epidemic Influenza," *Journal of the American Medical Association*, 72, no. 23 (1919): 1665–68.

82. MacLaughlin to Cumming, February 15, 1924.

83. Cumming to Graham, March 10, 1924.

84. Calvin Coolidge, "First Annual Message to Congress," December 6, 1923, retrieved from https://coolidgefoundation.org/resources/first-annual-message-to-the -congress/.

85. US Congress, *An Act to Limit the Immigration of Aliens into the United States, and for Other Purposes* (1924 National Origins Act), 68th Congress, Session 1, chapter 190, H.R. 7995, Pub.L. 68-139, 43 Statutes-at-Large 53 (May 26, 1924).

86. In 1924 there were 315,587 immigrants processed through the Port of New York; by 1925, that number had fallen to 137,492. Rates fell sharply again beginning in 1931 to 63,392. Immigration rates in the 1930s averaged less than 34,000 each year, with a low of 12,944 in 1933. Data for total immigration through the Port of New York by year found in Unrau, *Historic Resource Study, Ellis Island-Statue of Liberty National Monument*, vol. 1 (Denver: US Department of the Interior National Park Service, 1984): 185–86.

87. Frederick A. Wallace to James J. Davis, October 5, 1921, as cited in Unrau, *Historic Resource Study*, vol. 2, 553.

88. *Annual Report of the Surgeon General of the Public Health Service of the United States, for the Fiscal Year 1925* (Washington, DC: Government Printing Office, 1925).

89. Elliot Wadsworth, "Report to the Secretary of the Treasury on the Work of the Public Health Service at Ellis Island in Connection with the Admission of Immigrants," September 21, 1923, Unrau Papers, box 8, series IV, folders 111–13, BHML-EI.

90. The "Red Scare" was triggered by fears of a Communist uprising in the United States following the Bolshevik Revolution in Russia. As cited in Daniel J. Walkowitz, "Ellis Island Redux: The Imperial Turn and the Race of Ethnicity," in *Contested Histories in Public Space: Memory, Race, and Nation*, ed. Daniel J. Walkowitz and Lisa Maya Knauer (Durham, NC: Duke University Press, 2009), 137.

91. "Aliens Apprehended, Deported, and Required to Depart from the United States: 1892–1954," in Unrau, *Historic Resource Study*, vol. 1, 205.

92. *Report of the Ellis Island Committee* (New York: Department of Labor, 1934), 12.

93. Guthrie to Surgeon General, July 28, 1937, as cited in Harlan D. Unrau, *Historic Resource Study, Ellis Island, Statue of Liberty National Monument New York–New Jersey*, vol. 3 (Denver: US Department of the Interior National Park Service, 1984), 962–63.

94. *Annual Report of the Surgeon General of the Public Health Service of the United States, for the Fiscal Year 1923* (Washington, DC: Government Printing Office, 1923), 183.

95. *Annual Report of the Surgeon General 1923*, 183.

96. Sir Auckland Geddes, "Dispatch from H. M. Ambassador at Washington Reporting on Conditions at Ellis Island Immigration Station," London 1923, as cited in Unrau, *Historic Resource Study*, vol. 2, 568.

97. US Congress, *An Act in Amendment to the Various Acts Relative to Immigration and the Importation of Aliens under Contract or Agreement to Perform Labor* (1891 Immigration Act), 51st Congress, Session 2, chapter 551, 26 Statutes-at-Large 1084 (March 3, 1891).

98. US Congress, 1891 Immigration Act.

99. US Congress, Immigration Act of 1907; and US Congress, *An Act to Regulate the Immigration of Aliens to, and the Residence of Aliens in, the United States* (1917 Immigration Act), 64th Congress, H.R. 10382, Pub.L301, 39 Statutes-at-Large 874 (February 5, 1917).

100. "Dr. Jordan on Eugenics," *Daily Progress* (Charlottesville, VA), January 16, 1913, as cited in Gregory Michael Dorr, "Segregation's Science: The American Eugenics Movement and Virginia, 1900–1980" (PhD diss., University of Virginia, 2000), 2.

101. William Williams, "The Invasion of the Unfit," *Medical Record* 82, no. 24 (December 14, 1912): 1080.

102. *Book of Instructions for the Medical Inspection of Immigrants* (Washington, DC: Government Printing Office, 1903), 9–10.

103. *Regulations Governing the Medical Inspection of Immigrants* (Washington, DC: Government Printing Office, 1917), 20.

104. *Regulations Governing the Medical Inspection of Immigrants*, 20.

105. The intelligence test used at Ellis Island was adapted by Henry H. Goddard from an original test by Alfred Binet. In 1913 Goddard used his test on 152 immigrants, and his results indicated that more than 80 percent of them scored below the mental age of twelve; embarrassed by the biased findings, he "corrected" the data but still published results suggesting that more than half of immigrant arrivals were "morons." Skeptical

of the potential for bias in Goddard's test, USPHS physicians Howard A. Knox and Eugene H. Mullan instituted form boards and block puzzle tests to screen arrivals. See Alan M. Kraut, *Silent Travelers: Germs, Genes, and the "Immigrant Menace"* (New York: Basic Books, 1994), 74–75; and John T. E. Richardson, *Howard Andrew Knox: Pioneer of Intelligence Testing at Ellis Island* (New York: Columbia University Press, 2011), 97–141.

106. Robert Watchorn to F. P. Sargent, December 1, 1905, Unrau Papers, box 3, series IIIB, folder 36, BHML-EI.

107. *Annual Report of the Surgeon-General of the Public Health and Marine Hospital Service of the United States, for the Fiscal Year 1905* (Washington, DC: Government Printing Office, 1906), 274.

108. Robert Watchorn to F. P. Sargent, June 11, 1906, as cited in Unrau, *Historic Resource Study*, vol. 2, 597.

109. Unrau, *Historic Structure Report*, 448.

110. "Memorandum for Psychopathic Wards, 1922–24," as cited in Unrau, *Historic Resource Study*, vol. 2, 730.

111. "Memorandum for Psychopathic Wards, 1922–24," 730.

112. "Memorandum for Psychopathic Wards, 1922–24," 730.

113. Haskell, "Synopsis for the Guidance of Hospital Inspectors."

114. Daly, "Untitled notes," 1.

115. Daly, "Untitled notes," 1.

116. Acting chief medical officer E. K. Sprague, "Charges: Preferred against Miss Anna M. Brady, Attendant and Acting Nurse, by the Executive Officer of this Hospital," October 27, 1915, General records, Records of the Immigration and Naturalization Service, Record Group 85 (hereafter RG 85), National Archives Building, Washington, DC (hereafter NAB). The letter lists USPHS Order No. 48, regulating that all nurses remain on their assigned wards at all times while on duty.

117. *Regulations Governing the Medical Inspection of Immigrants*, 41.

118. Haskell, "Synopsis for the Guidance of Hospital Inspectors."

119. Haskell, "Synopsis for the Guidance of Hospital Inspectors."

120. Surgeon General Rupert Blue to Representative Thomas L. Reilly, November 1, 1915.

121. USPHS surgeon E. K. Sprague, "Examination of Attendant and Acting Nurse Anna M. Brady," October 27, 1915, General records, RG 85, NAB.

122. Sprague, "Examination of Anna M. Brady."

123. Sprague, "Examination of Anna M. Brady."

124. Sprague, "Examination of Anna M. Brady."

125. Surgeon General Rupert Blue to Dudley Field Malone, November 20, 1915, General records, RG 85, NAB.

126. Thomas W. Salmon, *The Care and Treatment of Mental Diseases and War Neuroses ("Shell Shock") in the British Army* (New York: War Work Committee of the National Committee for Mental Hygiene, 1917), 1–10.

127. J. D. Reichard, "A Neuropsychiatric Service in a Marine Hospital: Review of One Year's Work of the Clinic at Ellis Island," *Public Health Reports* 48 (September 15, 1933): 1137.

128. Reichard, "Neuropsychiatric Service," 1137.

129. Reichard, "Neuropsychiatric Service," 1137.

130. Reichard, "Neuropsychiatric Service," 1141.

131. Harriet Bailey, *Nursing Mental Diseases* (New York: Macmillan, 1936), 212–13.

132. Haskell, "Synopsis for the Guidance of Hospital Inspectors," 28; and Bailey, *Nursing Mental Diseases*, 223–35.

133. Reichard, "Neuropsychiatric Service," 1143.

134. Thomas M. Daniel, "The History of Tuberculosis," *Respiratory Medicine 100* (2006): 1862–70; and Barron H. Lerner, "New York City's Tuberculosis Control Efforts: The Historical Limitations of the 'War on Consumption,'" *American Journal of Public Health* 83, no. 5 (1993): 758–66.

135. John F. Murray, Dean E. Schraufnagel, and Philip C. Hopewell, "Treatment of Tuberculosis: A Historical Perspective," *Annals of the American Thoracic Society* 12, no. 12 (2007): 1749–59.

136. Any immigrant found to be suffering from TB in any form within the first five years of his or her arrival could be issued a warrant in violation of federal law and be subject to a deportation hearing with the Board of Immigration. Identification of these potential warrant cases was made easier through a broad screening campaign and mandatory TB reporting laws initiated by the New York City Health Department in the early twentieth century. "Notice, April 30, 1904, William Williams, Commissioner," as cited in Unrau, *Historic Resource Study*, vol. 2, 232.

137. J. G. Wilson, "Infectious Diseases of Children: A Study of 6,078 Cases among Immigrants with Special Reference to Cross Infection and Hospital Management," *Public Health Bulletin 95* (October 1918): 8; and Dispatch from H. M. Ambassador at Washington, "Reporting on Conditions at Ellis Island Immigration Station," London, 1923, as cited in Unrau, *Historic Resource Study*, vol. 2, 568.

138. Hugh S. Cumming, "Tuberculosis among the Ex-Service Men: With Special Reference to Its Bearing on Public Health," *Public Health Reports* 37 (September 15, 1922): 2241–52.

139. "Ward Use and Capacity, U.S. Marine Hospital #43, Ellis Island, New York, January 1924," from McLaughlin to Surgeon General, January 30, 1924, as cited in Unrau, *Historic Resource Study*, vol. 2, 640.

140. "Ward Use and Capacity," 640.

141. Cumming, "Tuberculosis among the Ex-Service Men," 2241–52. Detailed description of specialty treatment offerings (referred to as "Reconstruction Activities") on Ellis Island can be found in the "Synopsis for the Guidance of Hospital Inspectors" reports sent by the USPHS senior surgeon on Ellis Island in 1922, 1923, and 1924, Unrau Papers, box 8, series IV, folder 113, BHML-EI.

142. Arlene W. Keeling, "Organization and Innovation in the Early 20th Century," in Keeling, Hehman, and Kirchgessner, *History of Professional Nursing in the United States*, 144–46; and Jessica M. Robbins, "Class Struggles in the Tubercular World: Nurses, Patients, and Physicians, 1903–1915," *Bulletin of the History of Medicine* 71, no. 3 (1997): 415.

143. W. H. Slaughter, "Memo for the Handling of Patients Afflicted with T.B.," Unrau Papers, box 8, series IV, folder 113, BHML-EI.

144. Slaughter, "Memo for the Handling of Patients."

145. Slaughter, "Memo for the Handling of Patients."

146. Slaughter, "Memo for the Handling of Patients."

147. Slaughter, "Memo for the Handling of Patients."

148. Slaughter, "Memo for the Handling of Patients."

149. Slaughter, "Memo for the Handling of Patients."

150. A. Fergusen, USPHS acting assistant surgeon, memorandum for chief medical officer, May 25, 1936, Official Personnel Folder (hereafter OPF) of Margaret Veronica Daly, NPRC.

151. A. E. Brake, Chief of Personnel Records to the Secretary of the Treasury, July 9, 1936, OPF of Margaret Veronica Daly, NPRC.

152. "Summary of Hospital Transactions, U.S. Marine Hospital, Ellis Island, N.Y. for the Fiscal Year ending June 30, 1937," as cited in Unrau, *Historic Resource Study*, vol. 3, 965.

153. Gaston to Secretary of Labor, September 29, 1939, as cited in Unrau, *Historic Resource Study*, vol. 3, 822.

CHAPTER 6

1. Kathleen Dyer Hamm, oral interview with Paul Siegrist, September 11, 1991, courtesy the Statue of Liberty–Ellis Island Foundation, Inc., Ellis Island Oral History Project. Kathleen Mary Dyer Hamm was a nurse stationed on Ellis Island during WW2, from 1943–44. Author's poetic license for telegram.

2. Hamm interview.

3. Hamm interview.

4. Hamm interview.

5. "Entire City Put on War Footing: Japanese Rounded Up by FBI, Sent to Ellis Island— Vital Services Are Guarded," *New York Times*, December 8, 1941.

6. Arthur Dickson, oral interview with Paul Siegrist, June 30, 1993, courtesy the Statue of Liberty–Ellis Island Foundation, Inc., Ellis Island Oral History Project.

7. Anna Pegler-Gordon, "New York Has a Concentration Camp of Its Own: Japanese Confinement on Ellis Island during World War II," *Journal of Asian American Studies* 20, no. 3 (October 2017): 373–404. See also Clair Price, "Harbor Camp for Enemy Aliens," *New York Times Sunday Magazine*, January 25, 1942, 29.

8. Pegler-Gordon, "New York Has a Concentration Camp," 379.

9. Jeffrey Burton, Mary Farrell, Florence Lord, and Richard Lord, in "Confinement and Ethnicity," in *Department of Justice and US Army Facilities* (National Park Service, 1999): n.p., accessed from https://www.nps.gov/parkhistory/online_books /anthropology74/ce17a.htm; see also "Entire City Put on War Footing," 2.

10. Pegler-Gordon, "New York Has a Concentration Camp," 388.

11. "News about Nursing," *American Journal of Nursing* 42, no. 1 (January 1942): 115.

12. "News about Nursing," *American Journal of Nursing* 42, no. 3 (March 1942): 338.

13. "News about Nursing," *American Journal of Nursing* 42, no. 3 (March 1942): 338.

14. "News of Nursing," *American Journal of Nursing* 43, no. 1 (January 1943): 120.

15. "News about Nursing," *American Journal of Nursing* 43, no. 2 (February 1943): 230; "News about Nursing," *American Journal of Nursing* 43, no. 3 (March 1943): 320; and "News about Nursing," *American Journal of Nursing* 43, no. 4 (April 1943).

16. "News from USPHS—New Appointments," *American Journal of Nursing* 43, no. 5 (May 1943): 516.

17. "News from the USPHS," *American Journal of Nursing* 43, no. 9 (1943): 868; "News from the USPHS," *American Journal of Nursing* 43, no. 10 (1943): 965; "News from the USPHS," *American Journal of Nursing* 43, no. 11 (1943): 1054–55.

18. "Highlights of the Harbor: Shipyards Turnstile Tours," *Turnstile Tours*, accessed August 17, 2022, https://turnstiletours.com.

19. Hamm interview.

20. Hamm interview.

21. Arlene Keeling, observations during a personal tour of the hospitals of Ellis Island, March 8, 2017.

22. Ina Delaney, oral interview with Paul Siegrist, July 3, 1994, courtesy the Statue of Liberty–Ellis Island Foundation, Inc., Ellis Island Oral History Project. Delaney was a nurse stationed on Ellis Island from Spring 1943 through February 1944.

23. *Bill of Fare for the Immigrant Dining Room*, General History Box, Ellis Island Archives.

24. Hamm interview.

25. Delaney interview.

26. Erst Kerkhof, *Declassified Report of Ellis Island Camp*, October 21, 1944, 1–2. See also Werner Bubb and Van Arsdale Turner, "Report on Ellis Island Immigration Facility," March 29, 1946, 1–9, Inspection Reports on War Relocation Centers, 1942–1946, box 20, DECLASSIFIED—NND893002, General Records of the Department of State, Record Group 59, National Archives at College Park, MD.

27. Hamm interview.

28. Delaney interview.

29. Delaney interview.

30. Robert Funston and Carmelita Calderwood, *Orthopedic Nursing* (St. Louis, MO: C. V. Mosby, 1943): 42–57.

31. Funston and Calderwood, *Orthopedic Nursing*, 57.

32. Hamm interview.

33. John Parascandola, "John Mahoney and the Introduction of Penicillin to Treat Syphilis," *Pharmacy in History* 43, no. 1 (2001): 3–13.

34. Margaret Sandelowski, "The Physician's Eyes: American Nursing and the Diagnostic Revolution in Medicine," *Nursing History Review* 8 (2000): 3–38; see also Isaac Cox, oral history interview with Marcy Cohen, August 28, 1986, courtesy the Statue of Liberty–Ellis Island Foundation, Inc., Ellis Island Oral History Project.

35. Cox interview.

36. Cox interview.

37. Arlene Keeling, "Nursing in World War II: Overseas and at Home," in *History of Professional Nursing in the United States*, ed. Arlene Keeling, Michelle Hehman, and John Kirchgessner (New York: Springer, 2018), 257–83.

38. "History of Nursing in the USPHS," Commissioned Corps of the US Public Health Service, accessed March 3, 2022, https://dcp.psc.gov/OSG/Nurse/nrm-chapter-2 .aspx.

39. Thelma Robinson and Paulie Perry, eds., *Cadet Nurse Stories: The Call for and Response of Women during World War II* (Indianapolis, IN: Center Nursing Publishing, 2001), 173–85.

40. Keeling, "Nursing in World War II," 257–83; see also Federal Security Agency, "U.S. Marine Hospitals of the U.S. Public Health Service *Need* Senior Cadets," *U.S. Public Health Service NE Leaflet No.2*, accessed March 17, 2022, https://digirepo.nlm.nih.gov /ext/dw/101571902/PDF/101571902.pdf.

41. Burton E. Kane, oral history interview with Paul Siegrist, December 3, 1992, courtesy the Statue of Liberty–Ellis Island Foundation, Inc., Ellis Island Oral History Project. Dr. Burton Kane, a dental intern, spent May to September 1945 on Ellis Island and would later marry Nurse Irene Sabo.

42. Kane interview.

43. Eugenia K. Spalding, "The Senior Cadet Nurse," *American Journal of Nursing* 43, no. 8 (August 1943): 749–51.

44. Thelma Robinson, "Serving while Learning," in Robinson and Perry, *Cadet Nurse Stories*, 103–116.

45. R. D. Weiner and C. E. Coffey, "Electroconvulsive Therapy in the United States," *Psychopharmacolgic Bulletin* 27, no. 1 (1991): 9–15.

46. Robinson and Perry, *Cadet Nurse Stories*, 85.

47. Kane interview.

48. Louis Ford, oral interview with Debbie Dane, June 2, 1986, courtesy the Statue of Liberty–Ellis Island Foundation, Inc., Ellis Island Oral History Project. Louis Ford was a social worker on Ellis Island from 1948 to 1950 and recalled that immigrants were still coming and needed help with translation, finding relatives in different states, etc.; James Louis Baker, oral interview with Janet Levine, April 16, 1993, courtesy the Statue of Liberty–Ellis Island Foundation, Inc., Ellis Island Oral History Project. Dr. Baker also recalled that most of the patients during the years 1949 to 1951 were "merchant marine and coastguardsmen."

49. *Annual Reports of the Federal Security Agency, 1946–1949*, Records of the Public Health Service, Record Group 90, National Archives at College Park, MD.

50. "Proposes Closing of Ellis Island," *New York Times*, May 6, 1947.

51. (no first name) Zucker correspondence to District Director, May 9, 1949, Bob Hope Memorial Library, Archives and Special Collections, National Park Service at Ellis Island.

52. James Baker interview in Peter Coan, *Ellis Island Interviews: Immigrants Tell Their Stories in Their Own Words* (Denmark: Fall River Press, 2004), 3–4.

53. James Baker interview, *Ellis Island Interviews*, 3–4.

54. *Annual Report of the Immigration and Naturalization Service 1951*, 54–55, General records, Records of the Immigration and Naturalization Service, Record Group 85, National Archives Building, Washington, DC.

55. John Murray, Dean Schranfnagel, and Philip Hopewell, "Treatment of Tuberculosis," *Annals of the American Thoracic Society* 12, no. 12 (December 2015): 1749–59.

56. Oscar Ewins, quoted in the *New York Times*, December 28, 1950.

57. "Post-Peak Immigration Years, 1925–1954," National Parks Service, Ellis Island, accessed April 7, 2022, https://www.nps.gov/elis/learn/historyculture/places_post_peak.htm. See also "Ellis Island Ends Alien Processing," *New York Times*, November 13, 1954.

CONCLUSION

1. Barry Moreno, *The Illustrated Encyclopedia of Ellis Island* (New York: Barnes and Noble, 2010).

2. William Williams, as quoted in Lori Conway, *Forgotten Ellis Island: The Extraordinary Story of America's Immigrant Hospital* (New York: Harper Collins, 2007), 6.

3. Margaret V. Daly, "Nursing at Ellis Island: A Memoir," unpublished manuscript, n.d., typescript, 10, available at Bishop Hobbies, accessed October 16, 2019, https://www.bishophobbies.com/category/other-stuff/margaret-v-daly/.

INDEX

INDEX

ABOUT THE AUTHORS

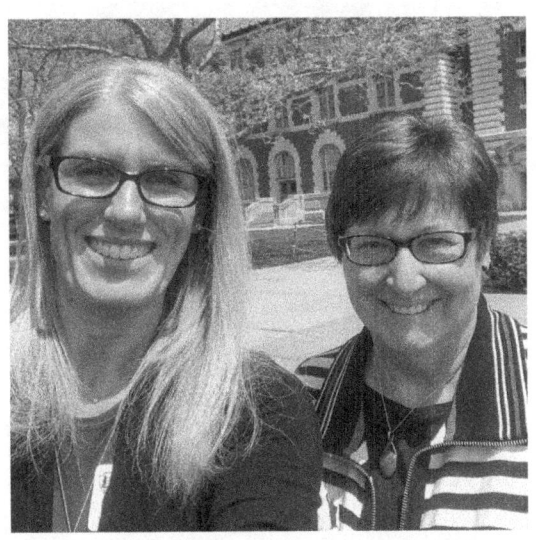

MICHELLE C. HEHMAN

Dr. Michelle C. Hehman is Chief Nurse Scientist at Nursing Science Partners and associate editor of *Nursing History Review*. An accomplished nurse historian, Dr. Hehman is also co-author of the award-winning textbook *History of Professional Nursing in the United States: Toward a Culture of Health*.

ARLENE W. KEELING

Dr. Arlene W. Keeling is the Centennial Distinguished Professor of Nursing Emerita at the University of Virginia School of Nursing. She is an award-winning author of numerous books, including *Nursing and the Privilege of Prescription* and *History of Professional Nursing in the United States: Toward a Culture of Health*.

Printed in the USA
CPSIA information can be obtained
at www.ICGtesting.com
CBHW030438011124
16730CB00007B/819